# Fundamentals of Health Care Improvement

## A Guide to Improving Your Patients' Care

THIRD EDITION

Gregory S. Ogrinc, MD, MS

Linda A. Headrick, MD, MS, FACP

Amy J. Barton, PhD, RN, FAAN, ANEF

Mary A. Dolansky, PhD, RN, FAAN

Wendy S. Madigosky, MD, MSPH

Rebecca S. (Suzie) Miltner, PhD, RN, CNL, NEA-BC

Foreword by Don Goldmann, MD

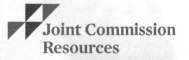
Joint Commission Resources

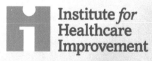
Institute *for* Healthcare Improvement

**Senior Editor:** Laura Hible
**Project Manager:** Allison Reese
**Associate Director, Publications:** Helen M. Fry, MA
**Associate Director, Production and Meeting Support:** Johanna Harris
**Executive Director, Global Publishing:** Catherine Chopp Hinckley, MA, PhD
**Joint Commission/Joint Commission Resources Reviewers:** Caroline Christensen, BS, Project Director and Certified Change Agent; Linda Faber, PhD, FACHE, Senior JCI Consultant

**Joint Commission Resources Mission**
The mission of Joint Commission Resources (JCR) is to continuously improve the safety and quality of health care in the United States and in the international community through the provision of education, publications, consultation, and evaluation services.

Joint Commission Resources, Inc. (JCR), a not-for-profit affiliate of The Joint Commission, has been designated by The Joint Commission to publish publications and multimedia products. JCR reproduces and distributes these materials under license from The Joint Commission.

The Institute for Healthcare Improvement (IHI) (www.IHI.org) is a leading innovator in health and health care improvement worldwide. An independent not-for-profit organization, IHI partners with visionaries, leaders, and frontline practitioners around the globe to spark bold, inventive ways to improve the health of individuals and populations. Recognized as an innovator, convener, trustworthy partner, and driver of results, IHI is the first place to turn for expertise, help, and encouragement for anyone, anywhere who wants to change health and health care profoundly for the better. Based in Boston, Massachusetts, with a staff of more than 140 people around the world, IHI mobilizes teams, organizations, and nations to envision and achieve a better health and health care future.

ISBN: 978-1-63585-037-6 (soft cover)
ISBN: 978-1-63585-038-3 (e-book)

For more information about Joint Commission Resources, please visit http://www.jcrinc.com.

# Contents

# Appendix: Tools to Help Your Improvement

# Dedications

For my friend Donel, who has shown exceptional courage and resilience. For Karen, my strength and love. — **GSO**

For Duncan Neuhauser and Paul Batalden, exceptional mentors and teachers of health care improvement. For David and Daniel Setzer, the heart of my life. — **LAH**

To Linda Cronenwett, PhD, RN, FAAN, for her exemplary transformation of nursing education and to the QSEN faculty and students who continue their improvement work on behalf of our patients. — **AJB**

To the interprofessional health care teams of the future for their commitment to not just do their work, but to also improve the systems in which they work. — **MAD**

With gratitude for my mentor, Linda Headrick, who leads and guides with purpose, and models integrity and lifelong learning. — **WSM**

To all the students and professionals who are continually learning how to make the health care system safe, timely, effective, efficient, equitable, and patient centered. — **RSM**

# Foreword to the third edition

We are in the midst of rapid—arguably revolutionary—changes in medical practice. When I was participating in epidemiological research in neonatal intensive care a few decades ago, very premature babies often died; now they almost always survive. As an infectious diseases specialist, I have seen HIV become a chronic disease, not a death sentence. I did not think I would see the day when hepatitis C could be cured by a course of oral therapy. Advances in genomics and precision medicine, treatment of cancer and chronic diseases, data analytics and machine learning, and technology are occurring at a dizzying pace. Thankfully, we are beginning to address the health of populations and communities rather than focusing so intently on acute care settings. Health care policy and payment are evolving to support the Triple Aim of improved population health, improved patient experience and outcomes, and controlled costs. The physician-dominated model of care is transitioning to team-based care, with increasing emphasis on the role of patients and families in shared decisions. Equity in health and health care remains a daunting challenge, especially in the United States, but there is growing consensus and increasing will to address persistent and unacceptable disparities in access, treatment, and outcomes.

How can caregivers prepare to incorporate these advances in their clinical practice? Translation of evidence into clinical practice always has been disappointingly slow, with enormous variation in the quality of care that patients experience. Speaking as a physician, I know that the young people I am teaching and mentoring will need to care for their patients far differently than I did when I was in training. Will they be ready to have a respectful conversation with their patients about the implications of a genetic testing result, the risk-benefit of a new cancer treatment protocol, or end-of-life care planning? Will they know how to address the social determinants and contextual factors that impact their patients' health and well-being? Or how to leverage technology and community services to keep frail elders safe in their homes?

Fortunately, there are scientific principles, methods, and tools that provide a foundation for meeting these challenges and improving the care of our patients. They are presented in a practical, readable format in *Fundamentals of Health Care Improvement: A Guide to Improving Your Patients' Care*. I am especially impressed by the book's rigor and emphasis on the scientific basis of improvement. This resource starts with an excellent review of the importance of evidence-based practice. I find that most students—and many career quality improvement specialists—have not been schooled in how to retrieve and weigh medical evidence. These skills are critical given the onslaught of bold claims for novel treatments and technologies, many of which have not been properly evaluated. These skills also are important in framing the pros and cons of therapeutic recommendations in discussions with patients and families in a way that they can understand. In my own practice, I have found that my efforts to engage my clinical and academic colleagues in improvement initiatives are far more effective when I start from a clear understanding of the evidence—including an honest assessment of the many practices for which evidence is missing or contradictory.

Improvement methods are presented with similar rigor, including a useful exploration of their underlying theories and conceptual models. For example, the chapter on team-based care leverages diverse sources and models to provide an explicit and practical approach to developing the competencies of team members and the team as a whole, as well as assessing team function. Fascinating historical examples, such as Florence Nightingale's polar-area diagram of preventable deaths in British soldiers, and Ernest Codman's end result approach to patient safety, enrich the text. Clinical vignettes are interspersed to give life and practical meaning to what otherwise might be pedantic summaries of the methods. The many informative diagrams, figures, and tables are succinct, clear, and literally could be "lifted off the page" and put into practice. In an era when clinicians tend to spend more time at the computer than at the bedside or talking to patients in the clinic, the book's emphasis on careful observation and rapid-cycle testing in partnership with patients is important and refreshing. The authors' blended, practical approach to teaching makes for an entertaining, engaging book.

I believe that this book will be a very useful and popular resource, not only for health and health care professionals in current practice, but especially for those in training. I am encouraged by the emphasis schools and training programs are placing on interprofessional learning and practice and their efforts to include improvement science in their curricula. Innovative approaches, such as the use of simulation in clinical settings and inclusion of trainees in health care system quality improvement initiatives, are promising. Health care professional schools, including a number of new medical schools, are immersing students in out-of-hospital prevention and care, as well as community and population health programs. Although a variety of resources can be tapped to help students begin their quality improvement journey, *Fundamentals of Health Care Improvement: A Guide to Improving Your Patients' Care* clearly demonstrates the added value of a well-crafted, practical book that is chock-full of methods and tools that can be applied immediately to improvement efforts regardless of their aim or setting.

Don Goldmann, MD
Chief Scientific Officer
Emeritus and Senior Fellow
Institute for Healthcare Improvement

# Foreword to the second edition

My sister asked me three questions, and I had no answers to them. These questions led me on a journey to think about how to improve the health care system. Although I was a staff nurse in an intensive care unit at the time, I began to see a new responsibility when I looked at the system through my sister's eyes. The responsibility to care for patients was familiar and rewarding, but I saw a new challenge: How could I improve the systems of care to ensure safer, more effective care?

The journey started when Robbie was just a few months old. Robbie was the first grandchild in my large family and was a happy, healthy, and adored child. When he was two months old, Robbie went to his pediatrician for his well-baby checkup; after declaring him in perfect health, his doctor advised my sister that he was going to administer Robbie's vaccinations. Shortly after returning home, Robbie was very ill, and my sister took him back to the pediatrician's office. He was transferred to an academic medical center and admitted to the ICU in respiratory distress. After a week in the hospital, Robbie was well enough to come home to his family, and he recovered completely over the following weeks.

At Robbie's four-month checkup, his doctor again told my sister that Robbie was in great health. As he proceeded to prepare the routine vaccination dose, my sister reminded him of what had happened after the two-month vaccination. The doctor paused and told my sister that Robbie's previous illness had not been a reaction to the vaccine. Despite her challenges, he assured her that Robbie would be fine but that he would administer only half the dose. He administered the vaccination, and Robbie died within 24 hours.

The questions my sister asked that changed my career were these: (1) How could the office and hospital patient records be so separated that the doctor couldn't see Robbie's whole journey? (2) How could the doctor not have known that a

half dose was the wrong treatment? and (3) Why didn't he listen to me?

These questions bring to the surface some of the problems in our health system today. Good practitioners struggle with broken systems and processes. Atul Gawande, a surgeon and best-selling author, has calculated that a physician interacting with a patient today has more than 13,000 possible diagnostic options and can prescribe from over 6,000 different medications. The complex journey of care requires new skills for all of us. It requires that we know how to, and do, deliver the best evidence-based care in accordance with an individual patient's circumstances and preferences and that we work cross-professionally to make the care system safer.

This book is your guide to becoming a complete health care professional, a strong caregiver, and an effective improver. The examples you'll study will be familiar, but the approaches to improvement may surprise you. By the end, you'll see the health care world with new eyes. You'll see systems in addition to symptoms. You'll think in daily PDSA cycles for improvement in addition to major change initiatives. And you'll see a new role for every health care professional.

Our patients rely on us to connect the pieces of the journey and to make it as safe as it can be. They rely on us to design and work within systems of evidence and with the knowledge supports we need. And they need us to listen.

Just five years ago, when I was teaching quality improvement methods to third-year medical students, I was rebuffed and heckled. "We have no power," they said. "Go call the CEO if you want things to improve." They recounted the challenges in their work with frustration and helplessness in their voices. They saw the problems in their daily work but saw no way out of the daily process failures. It's different today. In the few years since that depressing class, medical students, nursing students, and health professions students are building new skills in addition to the profession-specific knowledge they gain during their learning years. They know, now, not just what care to deliver but also how to improve the systems in which they deliver that care. Just three years ago, the Institute for Healthcare Improvement opened the IHI Open School for Health Professions (http://www.IHI.org/IHIOpenSchool) —a new way for students to build these crucial skills and to collaborate with other learners worldwide to improve care.

Here's an example of what makes me so optimistic today. Recently, three medical students met online through the IHI Open School virtual community and aligned their schedules to spend a month at IHI. They came and learned with our staff, met with experts from around the world, and began to improve safety in their earliest days of learning. They met Atul Gawande and studied operating room safety. They used WIHI—IHI's "radio station"—to teach fellow medical students throughout the world how to use surgical checklists. They collaborated to write a peer-reviewed article, "Check a Box. Save a Life: How Student Leadership Is Shaking Up Health Care and Driving a Revolution in Patient Safety" (http://www.ihi.org/offerings/ihiopenschool/resources/Pages/Publications/CheckaBoxSaveaLifeStudentLeadershipDrivingPatientSafety.aspx), and they developed an iPhone app to download the WHO Surgical Safety Checklist. These students have learned what you will learn in this book. You'll build a new way to see health care, from the patient to the system. You'll see the problems more clearly, and you'll see how to eliminate them. The skills you will build as you work through *Fundamentals of Health Care Improvement: A Guide to Improving Your Patients' Care* will make you a better clinician, a more valued team member, and will enrich your career as you serve the patients who rely on us for excellence.

Maureen Bisognano
President Emerita and Senior Fellow
Institute for Healthcare Improvement

# Foreword to the first edition

This book is about a better future: better outcomes for individual patients and populations of health care beneficiaries, better health care system performance, and better health care professional development—all linked together and in the lives of the people who will become tomorrow's doctors.

These doctors and their fellow young health professionals will
- Know that to be a professional and to be recognized as one, work will always have two aims: "to do your job and to improve your job."
- Be more than the naive system players of earlier times—they will know that every system is perfectly designed to get the results it gets—and that, therefore, their job goes beyond protecting their patients *from* the systems in which they work to being responsible for the design and redesign of those systems.
- Know that to achieve any sense of personal professional mastery, they must be involved in changing and improving the systems in which they work.
- Understand how measurement can be a friend of learning, redesign, and professional mastery and not just a tool for auditors, researchers, and payers.

This book is for them . . . and for those who seek to enable their futures. The basic knowledge and skills in this book can become the means of restoring a sense of "agency" in the health professionals of tomorrow. These skills will move advocacy into changed practices. Further, they will know that as professionals, they can use the systems they design and redesign to minimize the burden of illness—and from that knowledge will come a sense of mastery that will be deeply attractive.

Competence for a professional is always about knowing "that" something is so and knowing "how" something comes to be. Professional work is about performance: knowledge-in-action to meet the human need you face. In medicine, it is the interweaving of the science of disease biology and the science of clinical practice. Learning that interweaving and the professional work that flows from it is largely a matter of experiential learning—learning from doing and reflecting on it. This book is about that.

New information systems will enable a very different health care system. Information systems need accompanying process and system changes to make anything different occur. To do so will require attention to the material that is introduced in this book. This is likely to be a dynamic process, better considered in "verb forms" than in static "noun forms." Life in this world will be made more sensible by the topics introduced in this book.

These new professionals and their enabling faculty will enjoy the springboard from this book as together they will learn the lessons—the lessons that can only come by practicing and reflecting on that practice. Knowledge and skill for the redesign of care can come from the users of this book—learners and their teachers—actually engaging in tests of improvement and learning from them; but all improvement practice is practice, and to learn from it requires reflective review on the practice and its patterns.

Parker Palmer thinks that good teaching and learning often involve creating "space" within an idea, creating some working boundaries around the topic, and offering hospitality for the journey of discovery. Let your use of this book help you create that space for reflection, improvement, and learning.

The good news is that early signs show that professionals in the next generation of health care know they need to learn the material in this book and know they need to develop some skills in the application of the knowledge involved. They have seen the frustrations of those who have preceded them in the profession—frustrations about the prospect and reality of changing the practice and the context in which they work. Those in this new generation have grown up aware that the context for living is a world constantly re-creating itself. They want to take action on the gaps that can be seen. They value the agility that rapid-cycle tests of change rest on. This book and its tools and approaches can help them and their teachers together as this learning proceeds.

The authority of the authors of this book derives, in part, from their own generative "authoring" work in improving the quality of their own health care–giving and from what they have done to foster diverse learning environments that enable others to learn. In short, this book offers a great opportunity to learn, to practice, and to become a leader in tomorrow's health care system. Enjoy it.

Paul Batalden, MD
Professor Emeritus
The Dartmouth Institute for Health Policy and Clinical Practice
Dartmouth Medical School

# Introduction

*Fundamentals of Health Care Improvement: A Guide to Improving Your Patients' Care*, Third Edition, is designed for health professions students (medicine, nursing, pharmacy, and so on) and other health care professionals who are beginning to learn about clinical quality improvement. This book is intended to help health professional learners diagnose, measure, analyze, change, and lead systems improvement in health care. By applying these tools as well as the knowledge and skills you have acquired throughout your courses of study and training, you will learn how to create and shape reliable, high-quality systems of care for your patients.

In this third edition, we add the concept of coproduction of the improvement of health care services in partnership with patients, families, and communities. You'll notice that vignettes featured in the chapters focus on improvement opportunities and contain a patient on the improvement team. Patients and families are often the objects of improvement efforts, but improvement efforts are stronger and more lasting when patients, families, and communities coproduce outcomes with the health care professionals. The names of the clinicians and patients in the vignettes are fictional, as are the incidents. Any resemblance to actual persons, living or dead, or actual events is purely coincidental.

## Overview of Contents

This book provides nine informative chapters with relevant, timely content and updated figures, tables, and information. A new appendix offers a variety of engaging tools and resources.

## Chapter 1: Creating Teams to Close the Quality Gap

Chapter 1 explains the concept of a quality gap and describes ways in which health care can be improved through analysis of the quality gap. We present various models to further emphasize the importance of identifying gaps in health care and continuously working to improve patient care. This chapter also describes the positive outcomes that arise from productive teamwork and provides a set of criteria for identifying effective teamwork. In addition to learning how to assess factors that affect the way teams function, you'll learn the necessity of creating an improvement team of multiple health care professionals in partnership with patients and families.

## Chapter 2: Finding Scientific Evidence for Clinical Improvement

In Chapter 2 you will learn steps to take when collecting and evaluating evidence for the improvement of care. You will gain a clear understanding of the following: how to find evidence on the basis of a properly formulated question, how to evaluate the quality of evidence and research, and how to identify the most appropriate resources to use in finding evidence.

## Chapter 3: Identifying a Focus for Improvement

Chapter 3 offers valuable information on getting started with effective improvement work. After reading this chapter, you will be able to identify and focus on areas that need improvement. In addition, you will be able to organize your improvement goals by writing a clear aim statement.

## Chapter 4: Process Literacy and Systems in Health Care

In Chapter 4 you will learn the importance of describing the process of care as well as steps for choosing the most appropriate method for communicating about the process. Also included are instructions for considering the context and the organizational culture that influence clinical processes. After reading this chapter, you will know how to create an understandable, useful process model.

## Chapter 5: Measurement Part 1: Data Analysis for Decision Making in Health Care

Chapter 5 emphasizes the necessity of using data to improve health care and explains that different types of data are used to support different objectives. This chapter also discusses using a balanced set of measures for improvement work and introduces the value equation so you can identify a balanced set of measures for your improvement work.

## Chapter 6: Measurement Part 2: Using Run Charts and Statistical Process Control Charts to Gain Insight into Systems

In Chapter 6 we discuss the benefits of analyzing data over time so you can monitor the changes that occur in a system. Common-cause variation and special-cause variation are compared and contrasted in detail to provide an overview of what types of variation you might expect in a system. Examples of run charts and statistical process control charts help you understand the importance and benefits of displaying data over time.

## Chapter 7: Understanding and Making Changes in a System

Chapter 7 will help you manage complex system change and will show you how to identify barriers to change. In addition, we define complex adaptive systems and present several examples of Plan–Do–Study–Act (PDSA) to illustrate the testing and assessing of small cycles of change.

## Chapter 8: Spreading Improvements

Chapter 8 contains an in-depth case study of making and spreading change in a system. This chapter will enable you to identify strategies for sustaining and spreading change. As you read the practical, three-step approach for planning a successful spread effort, you will also learn how to overcome barriers to successful spread.

## Chapter 9: Publishing, Presenting, and Teaching Quality Improvement

In Chapter 9, we introduce you to the Standards for Quality Improvement Reporting Excellence (SQUIRE) publication guidelines. If you are interested in publishing your quality improvement work, this chapter will have the tips for you to be more successful in this endeavor. In addition, we provide a guide for educators by presenting four principles to develop educational experiences related to health care improvement and discussing the five stages of skill development in health care professionals. The chapter also has advice about how to evaluate your educational interventions.

## Appendix: Tools to Help Your Improvement

This appendix is new in the third edition and contains 16 tools that can be useful for doing and teaching improvement. These tools originated from Case Western Reserve University and the Institute for Healthcare Improvement. They range from an improvement project worksheet (that aligns with the content in this book) to skills for meetings to PDSA worksheets. Some of these worksheets augment and supplement material presented in this book. Other tools are presented as additional resources that may be helpful for you. Many of these tools are downloadable and adaptable to your organization; they can be accessed at https://www.jcrinc.com/assets/1/7/FHCI18_Tools_landing_page.pdf.

# Acknowledgments

The authors wish to acknowledge the time and effort of the following:

- Rachel Hammond, administrative assistant for Undergraduate Medical Education Affairs at the Geisel School of Medicine at Dartmouth, for her work in securing copyright permissions.

- Rebecca S. Graves, reference librarian at the University of Missouri Health Sciences Library, for her contributions to a prior version of Chapter 2.

- Pat Busick, MS, CIA, Iowa Lutheran Hospital, and Julie Gibbons, RN, BSN, CIC, Iowa Health Des Moines, for their willingness to share their story with us and for contributions to Chapter 8.

- Robert C. Lloyd, PhD, Executive Director, Performance Improvement, Institute for Healthcare Improvement, for his contribution to a prior version of Chapters 5 and 6.

- Marie W. Schall, MA, Senior Director, Institute for Healthcare Improvement, for her contribution to a prior version of Chapter 8.

- Tina Foster, MD, MPH, MS, Geisel School of Medicine at Dartmouth and Dartmouth-Hitchcock Medical Center, for contributions to the development of Chapter 9.

- Leslie Hall, MD, University of South Carolina School of Medicine, for contributions to the development of Chapter 9.

- Gail Armstrong, PhD, DNP, ACNS-BC, CNE, University of Colorado College of Nursing, for contributions to the development of Chapter 9.

- Paul Batalden, MD, Professor Emeritus, The Dartmouth Institute for Health Policy and Clinical Practice, Geisel School of Medicine, for providing an insightful review and an inspirational foreword to the first edition.

- Maureen Bisognano, President Emerita and Senior Fellow, Institute for Healthcare Improvement, for providing her graceful and thought-provoking foreword to the second edition.

In addition, Joint Commission Resources gratefully acknowledges the author team for the time, talents, and dedication each member wove into the third edition of this book. Special thanks to Don Goldmann, for his relevant, perceptive foreword to this edition. We also wish to express our appreciation to members of the Institute for Healthcare Improvement (Jane Roessner, Val Weber, and Marie Schall), as well as members of The Joint Commission and Joint Commission Resources staff (Cathy Hinckley, Helen Fry, Caroline Christensen, and Linda Faber), all of whom reviewed the manuscript and/or advised in its development.

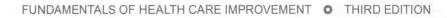

# Creating Teams to Close the Quality Gap

## Objectives

**After reading this chapter, you will be able to do the following:**

1. **Identify gaps in the quality of health care delivered to individuals and within the health system.**

2. **Identify members to be part of an interprofessional health care improvement team.**

3. **Describe how the Model for Improvement is used to help close the quality gap.**

"Every system is perfectly designed to get the results it gets."

—Paul Batalden, MD

## Improvement Opportunity

### Current Practices

Dorothy Baddour is a 65-year-old female who comes to the emergency department with a complaint of chest pain. Over the weekend, while working in her garden, she experienced several episodes of chest tightness, pain, and shortness of breath. Each of these episodes resolved itself, but this morning she had a much longer, more severe episode while carrying groceries up the stairs. The symptoms today were accompanied by cold sweats and aching arms. She called 911 and was taken to the emergency department at Regional Medical Center.

In the emergency department, Dorothy is cold and sweaty, and she appears ill. On physical examination, her lungs are clear to auscultation, and her heart has a regular rate and rhythm with a normal S1 and S2—no murmurs, gallops, or rubs. Her abdomen is flat and nontender. She has normal bowel sounds. There is no edema in her ankles.

# Diagnosing a Health System That Is Ill

For a straightforward case such as Dorothy's, most clinicians are comfortable identifying the major components of the history and physical exam. We also could identify additional elements:

- What is the patient's family history?
- Is she a smoker?
- Has she had a workup for chest pain in the past?
- Does she have high blood pressure?
- What is her pulse rate?
- Does she have jugular venous distention?

After reviewing the history and physical exam, a clinician might consider that this patient is experiencing an asthma attack, a heart attack, pneumonia, or perhaps gastroesophageal reflux. Many clinicians could identify diagnostic testing that should be done: an electrocardiogram, a chest x-ray, and likely some blood work.

In the scenario above, Dorothy is, in fact, having a heart attack—also called a myocardial infarction (MI). The clinical team proceeds to treatment options: administering an aspirin, oxygen, and a beta-blocker (medicine to slow down the heart rate, lower blood pressure, and decrease the work of the heart). Depending on the location and capacity of the hospital, the team might also arrange for the patient to have coronary angiography and angioplasty, with placement of a stent to open up her coronary artery. Another option would be to administer medications to break up the blood clot.

In health professions school, we train to evaluate and treat individual patients. In many ways, determining when a patient is ill is straightforward. We use knowledge and multiple skills: take a history, perform a physical exam, review diagnostic tests, confer with other health care professionals, and synthesize large amounts of data in order to provide evidence-based care for patients. However, it is more challenging to determine when a health care system is ill. Health professions students don't routinely learn how to assess, diagnose, and treat systems in health care. Think about this important question: How can you assess systems weaknesses and apply the resulting evidence to improve the quality of patient care?

> **" This book will help you, as a learner, diagnose gaps, identify measurements, enact changes, and analyze results, which will lead to system improvements in health care.**

This book will help you, as a learner, diagnose gaps, identify measurements, enact changes, and analyze results, which will lead to system improvements in health care. It provides the foundation of knowledge and skills specific to health care system improvement as well as exercises to develop these skills. Improving health care is a skill-based activity. In many ways, learning and practicing these skills requires effort that is similar to learning and practicing diagnostic and treatment skills; however, instead of an individual patient focus, the focus is on creating reliable systems of care that produce the highest quality for every patient, every time.

## Finding the Quality Gap

Examining outcomes of care is one way to identify when and where a system is broken. Let's focus on the use of beta-blockers as a treatment for acute MI and see if we can diagnose areas where the system is not working well. Figure 1-1 on page 13 shows data about the percentage of beta-blocker use after an MI. These are data from a classic research study that used a United States Medicare (federal health insurance plan that includes most individuals age 65 and older) database that is considered very useful for health system research. Published in 2000, the study compares outcomes of care for major teaching, minor teaching, and nonteaching hospitals.[1] The hospitals are stratified by number of resident physicians and number of hospital beds.

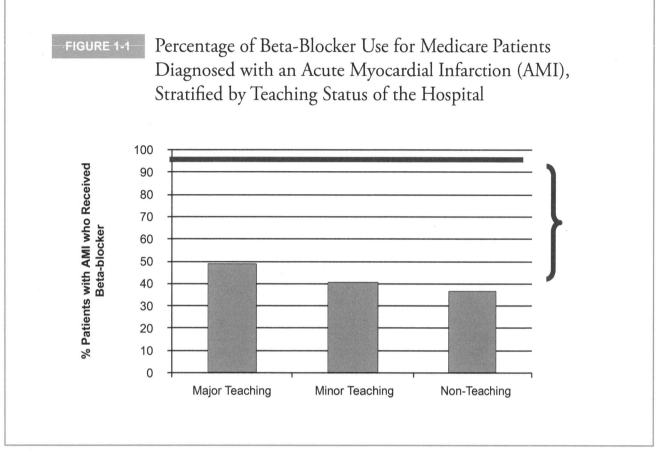

**FIGURE 1-1** Percentage of Beta-Blocker Use for Medicare Patients Diagnosed with an Acute Myocardial Infarction (AMI), Stratified by Teaching Status of the Hospital

The percentage of beta-blocker use for Medicare patients diagnosed with an AMI is stratified by teaching status of the hospital. This chart shows the quality gap between where the system is performing and where it should be performing.

One conclusion of the study was that major teaching hospitals provided better-quality care than did minor and nonteaching hospitals. As shown in Figure 1-1, major teaching hospitals prescribed beta-blockers 49% of the time, minor teaching hospitals 40% of the time, and nonteaching hospitals about 36% of the time. Although this study indicates that major teaching hospitals may provide better-quality MI care than minor and nonteaching hospitals do (these differences were statistically significant), the authors of the study note another important conclusion in their discussion: In the year 2000, patients such as Dorothy Baddour were receiving beta-blockers only 49% of the time at best.[1] Because beta-blockers are inexpensive, effective, and well tolerated, good-quality care dictates that the rate of use should be at least 95%—and probably closer to 100%. This difference between 49% and 95% is called the quality gap (*see* Figure 1-1, above). The quality gap is the difference between the expected level of care (95%

beta-blocker use) and the measured outcomes of a system (49%). These gaps in quality exist in all specialties and at all levels of the health care system.

Although this is a clear illustration of a quality gap, this study was published in 2000, using data from the late 1990s. Even though this specific quality gap has largely been closed in the United States, why was there such a large gap in 2000? The 2000 study uses data from the entire United States, so perhaps a snapshot of the system at a local level would give a different picture of how the system is performing. With this in mind, let's examine Figure 1-2 on page 14. The data in this figure are more recent (2017) and more local (although anonymous). We can assess beta-blocker use on several levels: Hospital 1 in 2017, Hospital 2 in 2017, and Dr. Jones's patients at the primary care Pine Tree Clinic in 2017. It is also possible to compare local performance to the top 10% in the United States and to the

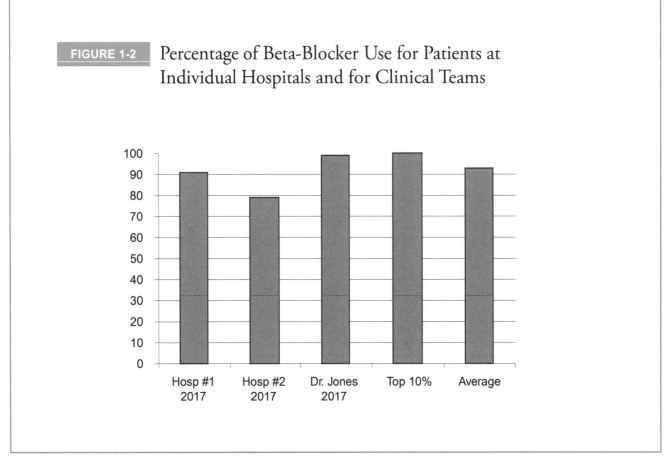

**FIGURE 1-2** Percentage of Beta-Blocker Use for Patients at Individual Hospitals and for Clinical Teams

The above chart illustrates comparative data for two hospitals, an individual provider, and the top 10% in the nation, as well as the national average.

national average. These local systems (that is, at the hospital level and clinic team level) were performing better in 2017 than were the systems in the 2000 study (*see* Figure 1-1, page 13). Why is this? Perhaps these hospitals and individual clinicians improved their skills over that period? Can we be sure that the quality gap that we recognized in 2000 is related to the systems of care and not just to clinician knowledge? Is there a way we can improve (diagnose and treat) the system so each patient gets the best care every time?

One possible explanation for the differences in beta-blocker use shown in Figures 1-1 and 1-2 is that the scientific data were not sufficient in 2000, and thus clinicians were not aware that using beta-blockers was the right treatment. Perhaps clinicians needed more scientific evidence that beta-blockers are an appropriate medicine to administer after an MI. As mentioned earlier, there are several undeniable conclusions about beta-blockers and MIs: Beta-blockers reduce mortality, are inexpensive, and are tolerated well. Data gleaned from a review of articles

(considered very strong evidence that has been summarized from many clinical trials) supporting beta-blocker use after MIs have been available since 1984.[2–5] Thus it is even more surprising that more than 50% of patients with acute MI were *not* receiving these medications in 2000—16 years later! More recently, research has shown that while the results of using beta-blockers for patients with acute MI improves mortality, appropriate dosing remains a challenge.[6] Surely electronic means of accessing information makes the dissemination of evidence-based practice easier, but the evidence alone is insufficient to change and improve systems of care.

## Evidence-Based Improvement

There is much more to putting evidence into practice than just having the right research evidence. The right evidence is often the focal point of most health professionals'

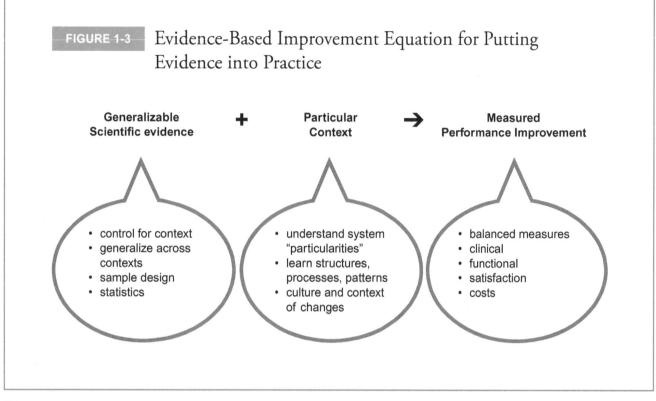

**FIGURE 1-3**  Evidence-Based Improvement Equation for Putting Evidence into Practice

| Generalizable Scientific evidence | + | Particular Context | → | Measured Performance Improvement |
|---|---|---|---|---|
| • control for context<br>• generalize across contexts<br>• sample design<br>• statistics | | • understand system "particularities"<br>• learn structures, processes, patterns<br>• culture and context of changes | | • balanced measures<br>• clinical<br>• functional<br>• satisfaction<br>• costs |

This equation demonstrates that generalizable scientific evidence must be applied within a specific health system to obtain measured performance improvement.

**Source:** Batalden PB, Davidoff F. What is "quality improvement" and how can it transform health care? *Qual Saf Health Care.* 2007 Feb;16:(1)2–3. Reprinted with permission from BMJ Publishing Group Limited.

education. Figure 1-3, above, is a model that shows the components of evidence-based improvement.[7] This model demonstrates how the best scientific evidence can be combined with knowledge of an individual system to produce improved outcomes for patients. The right-hand side shows that what we desire for our patients is *measured performance improvement*—for each individual patient and for our populations of patients. We want high-quality care for our patients in many domains: clinical, functional, satisfaction, and cost.

We often start with *generalizable scientific evidence* (*see* left-hand side of Figure 1-3, above). Generalizable scientific evidence comes from health care research in which investigators control for context and build knowledge that is generalizable across many contexts. This is where we use research design, carefully constructed methodology, and statistical analyses to evaluate treatments and therapies to determine the extent to which they are effective. As shown in the earlier beta-blocker example, 16 years after evidence

of the effectiveness of beta-blockers was known and widely disseminated in review articles, the treatment of patients with beta-blockers still lagged behind—even at academic medical centers.

## The Missing Connector

What's missing in health care is a connector—a set of knowledge and skills to take the best evidence and put it into practice consistently and reliably for the improvement of care for patients. The connector must take into account the particular context of the system being improved so we can understand the people, the existing processes, and the structure of the system. The people, processes, patterns, and structures are different between Hospital 1 and Hospital 2 in Figure 1-2 (page 14); therefore, the analysis of the system and the changes to improve the outcome will be different between Hospitals 1 and 2. The evidence about beta-blockers is the same, but the systems in which to incorporate that evidence are different. To improve care for patients, it's necessary to find the best evidence (in this case, that beta-blockers reduce mortality and morbidity after an MI) and link that evidence of best care with the specific knowledge of the local system providing that care (for example, use of computerized order entry, location of hospital, presence of an integrated cardiology unit).

## Caring for the System

Just as there are standard methods for assessing, diagnosing, and treating individual patients, an analogous set of tools exists for diagnosing and treating systems of care (*see* Table 1-1, page 17). For an individual patient, the clinician starts with a history and moves to a physical exam and diagnostic tests before arriving at a set of recommendations for therapy: comfort measures, medications, surgical interventions. Similarly, someone within a system (for example, a clinician such as yourself) often notices, through his or her own experience in the system or from discussions with others, that the system is not working well. Rather than just being frustrated by the system, clinicians can go on to the next phase of diagnosing the system, which may include creating process flow diagrams, reviewing outcomes data, or making fishbone diagrams. Finally, with a diagnosis and understanding of the system, the improvement team can recommend and test changes. Caring for a system is a natural extension of the skills that are used to care for individual patients.

 **Caring for a system is a natural extension of the skills that are used to care for individual patients.**

## Describing Improvement

The right-hand column in Table 1-1 describes the process of improvement in health care. There have been many terms (and many acronyms) used to describe improvement in health care: quality management (QM), total quality management (TQM), continuous quality improvement (CQI), systems-based practice (SBP), and practice-based learning and improvement (PBLI), to name a few. Performance improvement (PI) methodologies from other industries have also been applied to health care, including Lean, Six Sigma, and others. The largest US health care accrediting body, The Joint Commission (also the publisher of this book), requires health care organizations to engage in PI—not prescribing a particular methodology, although it does promote use of its own Robust Process Improvement® (RPI®) to help health care organizations move toward improved outcomes and high reliability (*see* Sidebar 1-1, on the right).

We realize that the alphabet soup of different quality improvement methodologies might be daunting, especially for students learning their particular health profession and now needing to understand another science—that of improving the care, treatment, and services that they provide. Although each of these performance improvement methodologies has nuances and roles in specific situations (for example, compliance, resident physician training, nursing education), we favor the more generic *quality improvement* and, even more simply, *improvement*, which incorporate aspects of many of these.

| SIDEBAR 1-1 | A Word About RPI |

The Joint Commission's performance improvement methodology, Robust Process Improvement, or RPI, combines data-driven problem-solving through Lean Six Sigma with the change management capability of Facilitating Change™. Facilitating Change is a set of actions, supported by a tool set, used to prepare an organization to seek, commit to, and accept change. The inclusion of change management emphasizes that more than a great technical solution is needed for sustainability. Recognizing the needs and ideas of the people who are part of the process—and who are charged with implementing and sustaining solutions—is key to building acceptance and accountability for system changes. Additionally, RPI helps interprofessional improvement teams pinpoint specific causes (for example, faulty maintenance procedures that do not keep hand gel dispensers full for hand hygiene) by identifying which practices are most prevalent in a particular microsystem. These tools then direct improvement efforts to eliminate the causes of failures. The Joint Commission's **Center for Transforming Healthcare (http://www.centerfortransforming healthcare.org/)** provides tools and additional information on using RPI to solve persistent health care quality and safety problems.

| TABLE 1-1 | Comparison of Diagnosing and Treating an Individual Patient Versus Analyzing and Improving the System of Health Care | |
|---|---|---|
| | **Individual Patient** | **System of Health Care** |
| **Initial Workup** | • Chart review<br>• History<br>• Physical examination | • Individual experience in the system<br>• Feedback from others in the system |
| **Further Workup** | • Blood work<br>• Laboratory tests<br>• Radiographs<br>• Functional tests | • Observation of the process<br>• Process flow diagrams<br>• Cause-and-effect diagrams<br>• Outcomes data |
| **Therapy/Treatment** | • Pain management<br>• Surgical intervention<br>• Medications<br>• Watchful waiting | • Model for Improvement<br>• Root cause analysis<br>• Plan–Do–Study–Act cycle |

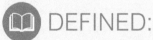 DEFINED:

### Quality Improvement

*Quality improvement* is best defined as the combined and unceasing efforts of everyone—healthcare professionals, patients and their families, researchers, payers, planners and educators—to make the changes that will lead to better patient outcomes (health), better system performance (care) and better professional development (learning).

Quality improvement is a shared responsibility.

*Quality improvement* is best defined as "the combined and unceasing efforts of everyone—healthcare professionals, patients and their families, researchers, payers, planners and educators—to make the changes that will lead to better patient outcomes (health), better system performance (care) and better professional development (learning)."[7(p.2)] This definition captures the focus of the three pillars of improvement (*see* Figure 1-4, page 18)—on health outcomes for patients, on performance of the health care system, and on the development of health care professionals. The inclusion of "everyone" in the center is key. Including everyone in this manner can have profound implications for an organization. For example, Walt Disney World, in Orlando, Florida, has a reputation for being impeccably neat and tidy; guests expect it to be so. A Disney executive, when asked how many people are on the cleanup crew, answered, "More than 45,000." He was not referring to an army of custodians, but to each and every person on the Disney payroll. Keeping the parks tidy is a priority for every person who works there. Similarly, the improvement of outcomes, systems, and professional development are foci for quality improvement for everyone from a new student to a practicing unit nurse to resident physicians, attending physicians, and chief nursing officers. Even patients and family members contribute to the three pillars. Quality improvement is a shared responsibility.

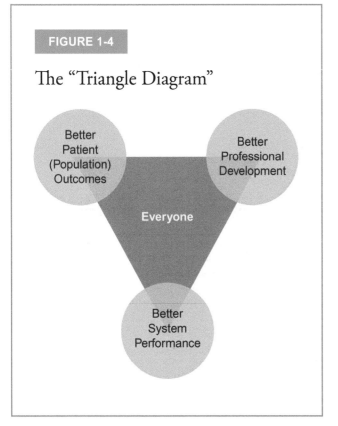

**FIGURE 1-4**

The "Triangle Diagram"

The three pillars of improvement—the system, the patient, and the professional—require everyone to be engaged in quality improvement

**Source:** Batalden PB, Davidoff F. What is "quality improvement" and how can it transform health care? *Qual Saf Health Care*. 2007 Feb;16(1):2–3. Adapted with permission from BMJ Publishing Group Limited.

## Relationships Among the Pillars

How are the pillars of the triangle diagram shown in Figure 1-4 related to one another? Consider an example of two leaders in an academic medical center. One leader, the vice president for nursing, has an advanced nursing degree and a master's degree in business administration. The other leader is the senior associate dean for education at the medical school and holds a medical degree. The vice president lives in the systems performance world, and her feet are firmly planted on the "better system performance" pillar. The education dean's feet are firmly planted on the "better professional development" pillar. Each of these individuals must recognize that the decisions and changes they recommend to the care system (or to the educational system) will also affect the other two pillars. In other words, even though his or her feet are planted on one of the pillars, the eyes and ears must recognize their close proximity to the other two pillars. The improvement of care is

interdependent on each of these elements. As a learner in the system, you also are a vital part of each of these pillars, and your efforts to improve the system of care will influence all of them. Thus, improvement is the professional responsibility of everyone in the health care system—and it depends on much more than just having the right scientific evidence at hand.

## Interprofessional teams for improvement

Teams and teamwork form the backbone of quality improvement work, and an interprofessional composition makes a team come to life. Although some may use the term *interdisciplinary* or even *multidisciplinary*, we favor the term *interprofessional*. The term *interdisciplinary* may be confusing because it can also mean cooperation between disciplines in a single field such as medicine; for example, pediatrics, surgery, and anesthesia are all disciplines within the field of medicine. Furthermore, the prefix *multi-* suggests that members can work independently toward a common goal, but the prefix *inter-* points to a collaborative effort.[8] Patients benefit from receiving care from a team of health professionals with expertise specific to their individual problems. With assistance from the patient as well as paraprofessionals, an interprofessional team provides a depth of knowledge and skills that surpasses the expertise of any one person.

## Improvement teams

Properly formed teams rely on the knowledge, skills, and experience of a wide range of people to solve problems. The dynamic interaction of the individuals helps them make good decisions and find effective solutions. But who are the members of an effective improvement team?

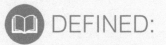 DEFINED:

**Improvement Team**
An *improvement team* should include the following members:

- System leader
- Team members with technical expertise
- Day-to-day leader(s)
- Executive sponsor
- Patient/family members

## System leader

An improvement team should include an individual with enough authority in the organization to institute a change. This person is the team's system leader; he or she understands the implications of the changes and can interact with other system leaders. The profession of the leader may vary based on the improvement activity. For example, if a group is working on improving the outcomes from coronary artery bypass graft surgery, a cardiothoracic surgeon might lead the improvement team. A team focusing on patient falls on the medicine wards might be led by a nurse leader who understands the local system and can advocate for interventions to reduce falls. A team working on reducing medication errors might be led by a pharmacist. Finally, patient flow issues such as discharge planning problems could be led by a health care administrator who understands the many levels of the discharge system and how the different clinicians come together at that point in time.

## Team members

Although these examples demonstrate who might be a reasonable leader depending on the focus of improvement, each improvement team represents an interprofessional effort involving individuals from multiple health care professions. The team needs members with technical expertise who understand the day-to-day workings of the system. These individuals across the professions understand how the systems operate and what an effective intervention strategy might include. An improvement project team also requires an individual for day-to-day leadership—someone who is part of the process on a daily basis. Another important addition to the team is an executive sponsor. This is an individual in a top management position with whom the team leader(s) has open communication. The executive sponsor is generally in a position to provide resources or remove barriers that the team may experience.

## Patients and families

Patients and family members are critical team members, as they provide unique insights into systems gaps and what possible changes may lead to improvements. Several attributes (listed in Table 1-2, below) contribute to engaging patients and family members in improvement teams.[9]

Involving patients and family members in health care improvement teams is only one aspect of engagement. Patients and family members can engage in health and health care at several levels (direct care, organizational design and governance, and policy making) as seen in Figure 1-5 on page 20.[10] Engagement is also a continuum from consultation (least engaged), to involvement (moderately engaged), to partnership and shared leadership (most engaged). In the case of improvement, patient and family member engagement is at the organization design and governance level and can exist across the continuum of engagement.

| TABLE 1-2 | Five Elements That Lead to Activating Patients, Families, and Professionals for the Coproduction of Improved Care |
|---|---|
| Readiness | Be ready mentally and emotionally to engage in improving care. |
| Curiosity | Ask questions and seek answers. |
| Reframe | Turn challenges into opportunities for learning and improvement. |
| Listen and Learn | Seek out new knowledge and ideas. |
| Participate | Be present and personally participate. |

**Source:** Sabadosa KA, Batalden PB. The interdependent roles of patients, families and professionals in cystic fibrosis: A system for the coproduction of health care and its improvement. *BMJ Qual Saf.* 2014 Apr;23 Suppl 1:i90–94. Reprinted with permission from BMJ Publishing Group Limited.

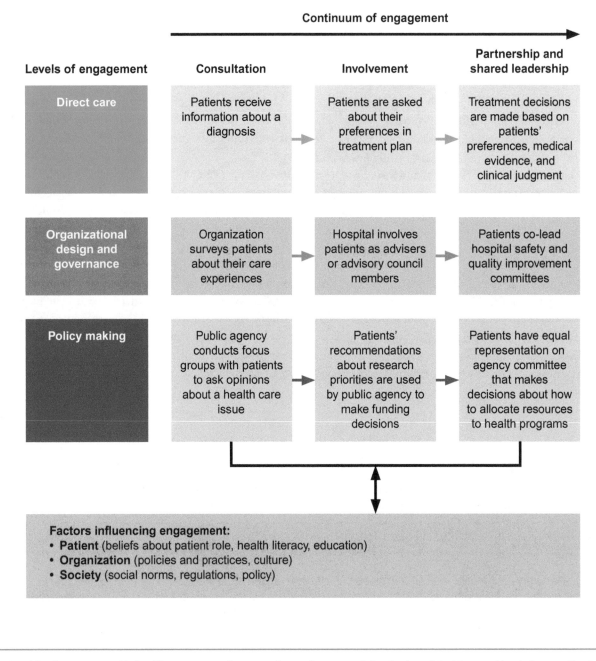

**FIGURE 1-5** A Multidimensional Framework for Patient and Family Engagement in Health and Health Care

Continuum of engagement

| Levels of engagement | Consultation | Involvement | Partnership and shared leadership |
|---|---|---|---|
| Direct care | Patients receive information about a diagnosis | Patients are asked about their preferences in treatment plan | Treatment decisions are made based on patients' preferences, medical evidence, and clinical judgment |
| Organizational design and governance | Organization surveys patients about their care experiences | Hospital involves patients as advisers or advisory council members | Patients co-lead hospital safety and quality improvement committees |
| Policy making | Public agency conducts focus groups with patients to ask opinions about a health care issue | Patients' recommendations about research priorities are used by public agency to make funding decisions | Patients have equal representation on agency committee that makes decisions about how to allocate resources to health programs |

**Factors influencing engagement:**
- **Patient** (beliefs about patient role, health literacy, education)
- **Organization** (policies and practices, culture)
- **Society** (social norms, regulations, policy)

Patient and family engagement in health care occurs along a continuum from consultation to shared decisions and leveled across the direct care situation to organizations and public policy.

**Source:** Carman KL, et al. Patient and family engagement: A framework for understanding the elements and developing interventions and policies. *Health Aff (Millwood)*. 2013 Feb;32(2):2223–2231. Reprinted with permission from Project HOPE/*Health Affairs*. www.healthaffairs.org.

As health care improvement becomes part and parcel of providing care, improvement activities will become a core function of interprofessional clinical teams including patients/family members.

# The Model for Improvement

Fortunately, a model exists for interprofessional clinical teams to connect our best-practice evidence with our local health care delivery system. The Model for Improvement (*see* Figure 1-6, right) provides a structure for diagnosing and treating systems of care.[11] The model is based on the work of W. Edward Deming and his theory, the System of Profound Knowledge, and is used by organizations such as the Institute for Healthcare Improvement and the Agency for Healthcare Research and Quality. There are, of course, other models that can be used for improvement work. As mentioned earlier, The Joint Commission created RPI, which blends concepts from Lean, Six Sigma, and change management methodologies.

We use the Model for Improvement throughout this book and return to it often as we delve deeper into the specific knowledge and skill components of clinical improvement. See Sidebar 1-2 on page 22 for information on additional models used to improve systems and processes.

Why do we believe that the Model for Improvement is effective? There are many examples in the literature of systems that have been improved with the methods proposed in this model. Clinicians have used this methodology to improve measurement of disability for pediatric patients experiencing chronic pain,[12] to improve care for patients with diabetes in a primary care clinic,[13] to reduce falls and injury from falls in hospitalized patients,[14] and to improve safety across sites within a health system.[15] Each of these represents an example of improving the system of care for patients. Across these examples there is one very consistent bottom line: *Improving health care is a contact sport*—it is something that we do. Improvement does *not* occur by simply attending a lecture, sitting in a meeting, reading a book (not even this book!), or performing online simulations. We achieve this improvement through experience in applying these methods, and this experience is necessary for achieving competence in the full range of skills needed for clinical practice.

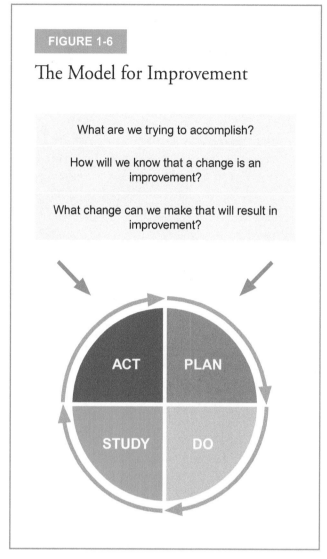

**FIGURE 1-6**

## The Model for Improvement

What are we trying to accomplish?

How will we know that a change is an improvement?

What change can we make that will result in improvement?

ACT · PLAN · STUDY · DO

This model suggests a basic approach to improvement work, based on the answers to three questions. It suggests that planned change, implementation and analysis of the change, and creation of a plan moving forward are key components of improvement work.

**Source:** Adapted from Langley GJ, et al. *The Improvement Guide: A Practical Approach to Enhancing Organizational Performance*, 2nd ed. San Francisco: Jossey-Bass, 2009. Printed with permission.

## Three questions in the Model for Improvement

If system improvement is a skill to learn and practice, how is it done? In this book, we focus on the widely used and easily available Model for Improvement. It is basic and simple to understand and use. The model distills the improvement process into three questions:

- What are we trying to accomplish? (aim)
- How will we know a change is an improvement? (measures)
- What change can we make that will result in improvement? (changes)

Quality Improvement Programs

A number of quality improvement (QI) programs exist in addition to the Model for Improvement that is highlighted in this book. We use the Model for Improvement because we believe it teaches foundational concepts and skills that are applicable to a wide variety of settings. It is basic and easy to understand for health care professions students and others. Organizations often choose one QI program so that there is consistency for faculty, staff, and learners in the organization. However, you may encounter—or may want to apply—one or more improvement programs in your health care organization. Each program described below can be considered the "next generation" of performance improvement, has strengths, and often has specific terminology.

**Six Sigma**
- Developed by Motorola and popularized by General Electric
- Goal is to achieve defect-free performance at the level of three or fewer defects per million (that is, six sigma)
- Steps are to recognize, define, measure, analyze, improve, control, standardize, integrate

**Lean**
- Developed by Toyota and known as the Toyota Production System
- Key theory is to reduce waste and increase speed
- Emphasis on work flow and customer orientation

**Lean Six Sigma**
- Five-step problem-solving approach (DMAIC—Define, Measure, Analyze, Improve, Control)
- Certification to designate expertise (Yellow, Green, and Black Belts)

**Robust Process Improvement (RPI)**
- Developed by The Joint Commission to improve system processes and clinical outcomes
- Blends Lean, Six Sigma, and change management methodologies
- Focuses on building expertise of staff and leadership, embedding tools and methods into everyday work
- Is key toward moving health care organizations to high reliability

Once we determine the answers to these three questions, we can use the Plan–Do–Study–Act (PDSA) cycle to design and test changes on a small scale. In this book, we will cover each of these steps in depth in subsequent chapters.

As an introduction to using the Model for Improvement to close a quality gap, let's return to the example of beta-blockers. In Figure 1-2, page 14, we see a beta-blocker quality gap of more than 20%. In Hospital 2 the leadership has formed a team to work on closing this beta-blocker quality gap. The beta-blocker after myocardial infarction (BAMI) team consists of the chief cardiology resident, a cardiac care nurse with training in quality improvement, a medical student, a pharmacist, the nurse discharge coordinator, and a patient who has had an MI.

**Creating the aim.** The BAMI team at Hospital 2 starts by creating an aim:

> "In the next six months, we will increase the rate of beta-blocker use in patients at discharge after MI to greater than 90%."

This is a strong, clear aim. It states who is going to be working on this aim, what they are going to be doing, what the exact goal is, and when the results should be achieved.

**Determining the measures.** After setting the aim, the BAMI team determines the measures it will use in judging the success of achieving the aim. For this example, the measure is relatively straightforward:

> "The percentage of MI patients who receive a beta-blocker at discharge from the hospital"

Because this is the same indicator that showed the gap in quality, monitoring this indicator (percentage of patients receiving beta-blockers) monthly will help determine whether progress is being made.

**Testing changes.** For possible changes, the BAMI team holds a brainstorming session to list how to change the system and ensure that every patient who has had an MI reliably receives a beta-blocker at discharge. As shown in Figure 1-7, on the right, the team is able to identify several possible interventions, including the following:
- Educate the physicians about the benefits of beta-blockers.
- Teach the patient and the family that beta-blockers are important to keep the heart healthy.
- Have the pharmacist review medications at discharge.
- Encourage nurses to identify beta-blockers at discharge.
- Generate a prescription for beta-blocker.

The BAMI team does not know which of these would be most effective, but by systematically trying each one (using the PDSA methodology), the team can test each intervention and measure its impact.

This brief example oversimplifies the improvement process; in truth, the aim, measures, and changes may take several weeks or months for the team to develop. Care delivery systems do not improve by chance; nor do they improve simply through the development of new knowledge. As indicated in the beta-blocker example, it took almost 20 years for knowledge about the benefits of beta-blockers to become embedded in health care systems and thus close the

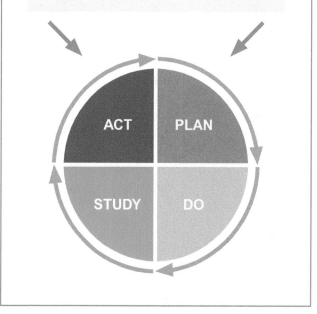

**FIGURE 1-7**

## The Beta-Blocker After Myocardial Infarction (BAMI) Improvement Team Worksheet

In the next six months, increase the rate of beta-blocker use in patients at discharge after a myocardial infarction to greater than 90%.

Measure the percentage of patients who have a myocardial infarction who receive a beta-blocker at discharge from the hospital.

Possible interventions:
1. Educate the physicians.
2. Educate the patient and family.
3. Have pharmacists review discharge meds.
4. Encourage nurses to identify beta-blockers at discharge.
5. Generate prescription for beta-blocker automatically and place it on the patient's chart.

ACT  PLAN
STUDY  DO

This worksheet applies the Model for Improvement to our beta-blocker case study.

**Source:** Adapted from Langley GJ, et al. *The Improvement Guide: A Practical Approach to Enhancing Organizational Performance*, 2nd ed. San Francisco: Jossey-Bass, 2009. Printed with permission.

quality gap (*see* Figures 1-1 and 1-2, pages 13 and 14). Quality improvement can accelerate the system changes needed to close those gaps.

# Summary

Quality gaps exist in all areas of health care: vaccination rates for children, treatment for patients with post-traumatic stress disorder, surgical wound infections, turnaround time for specimens sent to a pathology lab, follow-up of radiology tests, outpatient blood pressure control, and so on. Quality gaps affect every health care profession, every practice specialty, and potentially every patient. As health care professionals, we have a duty to improve the systems in which we work. Just as you learn to take a history, perform patient assessments and physical exams, and recommend and implement treatments for patients, you also must learn how to analyze and measure systems of care and recommend and implement system-level changes (*see* Table 1-1, page 17). Our job as health care professionals is not only to *provide* care but also to *improve* care.

Although this may seem a daunting task, you can learn the skills for improving patient care systems just as you learn the skills for providing pain management, drawing blood samples, auscultating the heart, or evaluating chest x-rays. This book walks you through the development of improvement skills. It shows you how to evaluate systems and apply changes to improve the delivery of care. This book will give you knowledge to view the clinical setting differently—through a "systems lens." After reading this book, you'll be able to identify how to measure clinical care in a comprehensive way that accounts for clinical outcomes, patient functional ability, patient and staff satisfaction, and even the costs of care. As clinical improvement becomes a routine part of clinical care, you'll be ready to recommend changes to systems that are embedded in the care system so that patients like Dorothy Baddour reliably receive the right care at the right time.

## Study Questions

1. What gaps have you seen in clinical care that might suggest a need for improvement?
2. What is your experience with teams engaged in improvement work?
3. How might you apply the Model for Improvement in a self-improvement activity related to healthy living or study habits?

## References

1. Allison JJ, et al. Relationship of hospital teaching status with quality of care and mortality for Medicare patients with acute MI. *JAMA*. 2000 Sep 13;284(10):1256–1262.

2. Hjalmarson A. Early intervention with a beta-blocking drug after acute myocardial infarction. *Am J Cardiol*. 1984 Dec 21;54(11):11E–13E.

3. Frishman WH, Ruggio J, Furberg C. Use of beta-adrenergic blocking agents after myocardial infarction. *Postgrad Med*. 1985 Dec;78(8):40–46, 49–53.

4. Davenport J, Whittaker K. Secondary prevention in elderly survivors of heart attacks. *Am Fam Physician*. 1988 Jul;38(1):216–224.

5. Hjalmarson A. International beta-blocker review in acute and postmyocardial infarction. *Am J Cardiol*. 1988 Jan 29;61(3):26B–29B.

6. Goldberger JJ, et al. Effect of beta-blocker cose on survival after acute myocardial infarction. *J Am Coll Cardiol*. 2015 Sep 29;66(13):1431–1441.

7. Batalden PB, Davidoff F. What is "quality improvement" and how can it transform healthcare? *Qual Saf Health Care*. 2007 Feb;16(1):2–3.

8. Bridges DR, et al. Interprofessional collaboration: Three best practice models of interprofessional education. *Med Educ Online*. 2011 Apr 8;16.

9. Sabadosa KA, Batalden PB. The interdependent roles of patients, families and professionals in cystic fibrosis: A system for the coproduction of healthcare and its improvement. *BMJ Qual Saf*. 2014 Apr;23 Suppl 1:i90–94.

10. Carman KL, et al. Patient and family engagement: A framework for understanding the elements and developing interventions and policies. *Health Aff (Millwood)*. 2013 Feb;32(2):2223–2231.

11. Langley GJ, et al. *The Improvement Guide: A Practical Approach to Enhancing Organizational Performance*, 2nd ed. San Francisco: Jossey-Bass, 2009.

12. Lynch-Jordan AM, et al. Applying quality improvement methods to implement a measurement system for chronic pain-related disability. *J Pediatr Psychol*. 2010 Jan–Feb;35(1):32–41.

13. Johnson P, Raterink G. Implementation of a diabetes clinic-in-a-clinic project in a family practice setting: Using the plan, do, study, act model. *J Clin Nurs*. 2009 Jul;18(14):2096–2103.

14. Neily J, et al. One-year follow-up after a collaborative breakthrough series on reducing falls and fall-related injuries. *Jt Comm J Qual Patient Saf*. 2005 May;31(5):275–285.

15. Dixon-Woods M, et al. *Safer Clinical Systems: Evaluation Findings. Learning from the Independent Evaluation of the Second Phase of the Safer Clinical Systems Programme*. London: The Health Foundation, 2015.

# Finding Scientific Evidence for Clinical Improvement

 Objectives

**After reading this chapter, you will be able to do the following:**

1. Describe the link between the best evidence and the system of care.
2. Recognize the range and depth of questions that should be asked to find supporting evidence for the improvement of care.
3. Recognize the relative strength of research evidence and the difference between filtered and unfiltered evidence.
4. Identify the proper use of resources—including electronic resources and reference librarians—to find evidence for health care improvement.

 Improvement Opportunity

## A Clinical Conundrum

A team of students from pharmacy, nursing, and medicine is awaiting the start of interprofessional rounds on a medical ward. As they wait, the students comment on today's cold winter weather and on the number of patients admitted with community-acquired pneumonia (CAP).

For the past two weeks, the attending has recommended that the team use a combination of ceftriaxone and azithromycin for empirical antibiotic treatment of CAP. Today there is a new attending, however, who insists that patients receive single coverage with levofloxacin. The new attending is adamant in stating that single antibiotic coverage is simple, appropriate, and evidence-based.

The students are confused. Why is the treatment protocol changing? Is it based on the individual preference of the new attending, or does evidence exist to support this approach? During lunch the students agree to meet at the library after their clinical shift to explore the evidence for treatment of CAP. As they scan the National Guideline Clearinghouse website (https://www.guideline.gov), the students come across the section on CAP (https://www.guideline.gov/summaries/summary/50009/pneumonia-in-adults-diagnosis-and-management?q=community+acquired+pneumonia).[1] This section includes several links to practice guidelines and position statements from professional organizations and is intended for use by nurses, pharmacists, physicians, advanced practice nurses, physician assistants, and all health care professions.

Each student reviews the guideline.gov information, but then also looks at specific recommendations from other organizations. The pharmacy student chooses the Infectious

Diseases Society of America link and finds that it contains extensive, exhaustively cited information.[2] It is also from 2007 with a note that it is currently being updated in 2017. She has neither the time nor the inclination to read it all, so she moves to the table of summary recommendations. She is a bit surprised to find that empirical treatment for CAP is acceptable with either a combination of third-generation cephalosporin (ceftriaxone) and an advanced macrolide (azithromycin) or with a single agent such as a fluoroquinolone (levofloxacin). When she relays this to the nursing and medical students, they, too, are puzzled and even a bit dismayed. The students understand the

microbiology and pharmacology behind either the antibiotic combination or the individual antibiotic as acceptable empirical coverage for likely causes of CAP; however, these guidelines are confusing to them.

With something as straightforward as antibiotics for a rather common infection, how is one to decide which is the right recommendation to follow? Both recommendations are supported by reams of research, but is one more correct than the other? Can both be right? Might the patient have a preference, or the insurance coverage guide a decision?

# The Importance of Evidence-Based Practice

The use of evidence in health care has grown logarithmically in recent years. New scientific knowledge is generated by researchers, scholars, and clinicians at a rate of more than 10,000 articles per year. The amount and the configuration of data and information can be overwhelming. Since the notion and use of *evidence-based practice* (EBP) for clinical decision-making became prominent in the 1990s,[3–7] the discipline of managing and using evidence has continued to grow.

EBP is "the process of shared decision-making between practitioner, patient, and others significant to them based on research evidence, the patient's experience and preferences, clinical expertise or know-how, and other available robust sources of information."[4(p. 57)] At the University of Colorado Hospital, this definition of EBP has evolved into health professionals' practice of placing the patient at the center of the practice model, surrounded by sources of evidence and supported by organizational infrastructure (*see* Figure 2-1, page 27).[5] At the core of the model is the patient and his or her preferences, values, and experiences. Valid and current research provides the best evidence for the situation.

## Sources Beyond Research

When research evidence is limited or inconclusive, the model identifies eight additional sources of evidence to help inform care:

1. Pathophysiology
2. Retrospective or concurrent medical record review
3. Quality improvement and risk data
4. International, national, and local standards
5. Infection control data
6. Clinical expertise
7. Benchmarking data
8. Cost-effectiveness analysis

EBP involves applying the best-known evidence using the clinician's judgment for an individual patient at a point in time. Clinicians do not consider any one of these sources of evidence as more important than another, although a particular decision may require giving more weight to one element than another. For example, a patient who is a Jehovah's Witness may meet all the criteria for a red blood cell transfusion; however, because of the patient's preferences, clinicians will not give the patient blood products. True application of EBP involves bringing patient preferences, experience, and values along with valid research and additional sources of evidence to bear on patient care decisions.

## Limitations of EBP

Over the past several years, EBP has begun to show some of the limitations in its methodological ability to improve care and outcomes for patients. Because there is an abundance of evidence available, finding it is usually not an issue. In the example of beta-blocker prescribing after myocardial infarction in Chapter 1, we saw that although strong evidence had been readily available in the published

FIGURE 2-1 The Colorado Patient-Centered Interprofessional Evidence-Based Practice Model

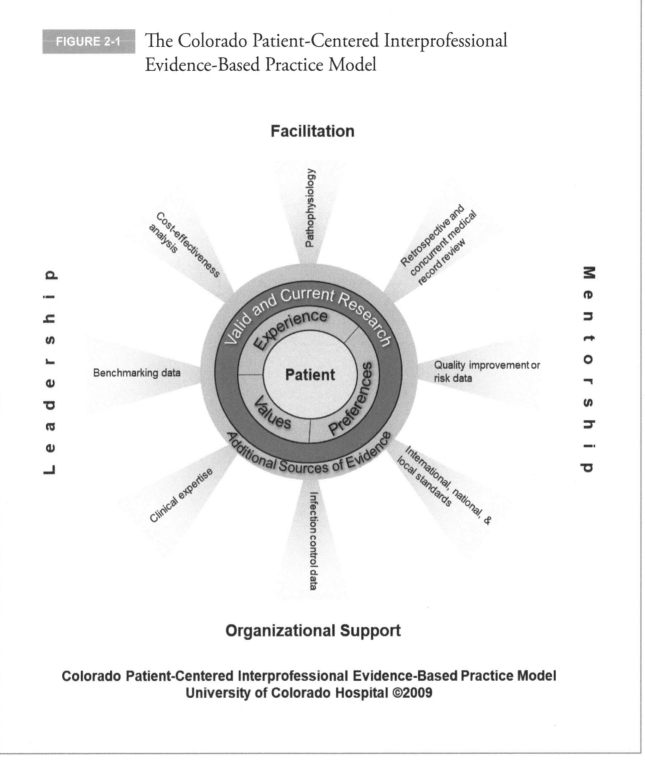

One model of evidence-based practice from University of Colorado Hospital. Notice the patient at the center and the multiple components feeding the use of evidence in practice.

**Source:** Goode CJ, et al. The Colorado Patient-Centered Interprofessional Evidence-Based Practice Model: A framework for transformation. *Worldviews Evid Based Nurs.* 2010 Dec;8(2):96–105. Reprinted with permission.

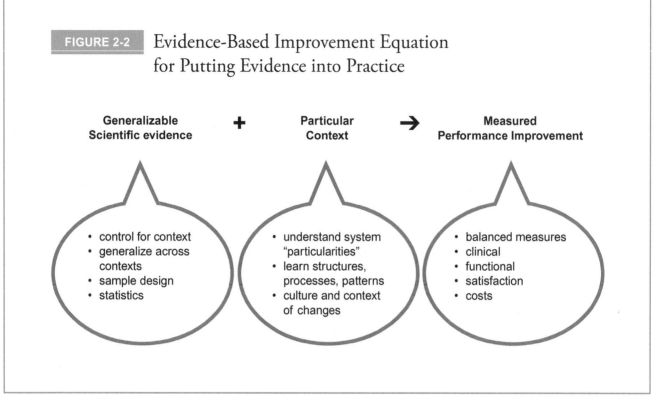

**FIGURE 2-2** Evidence-Based Improvement Equation for Putting Evidence into Practice

Generalizable Scientific evidence **+** Particular Context **→** Measured Performance Improvement

- control for context
- generalize across contexts
- sample design
- statistics

- understand system "particularities"
- learn structures, processes, patterns
- culture and context of changes

- balanced measures
- clinical
- functional
- satisfaction
- costs

The evidence-based improvement equation must be applied within a specific health system to obtain measured performance improvement.

**Source:** Batalden PB, Davidoff F. What is "quality improvement" and how can it transform health care? *Qual Saf Health Care.* 2007 Feb;16:(1)2–3. Reprinted with permission from BMJ Publishing Group Limited.

literature for more than 15 years, the data had not made a full impact on practice (fewer than 50% of patients received this treatment). As the students discovered in the opening vignette, finding the evidence is the first step. They must then interpret and apply it to a specific patient encounter. Health care professionals are awash in evidence that is prepackaged into guidelines and reviews. Not all diagnostic and therapeutic situations are backed by evidence, but for those that are (for example, treatment of diabetes, timing of perioperative antibiotics, prenatal testing, and many others), application of the evidence in practice can be irregular and inconsistent.

## Linking evidence to systems of care

Although guidelines might be explicit, the application of this knowledge locally is implicit and based on the local practice patterns in a setting.[6] Simply making the knowledge available does not reliably bridge the gaps in care for populations of patients.[7] EBP emphasizes applying evidence to one patient at a time, but this limits its impact if the best evidence is not connected to care for all patients in a specific system or context. EBP provides a solid

foundation for asking the right questions and finding answers to apply to patient care; however, it is limited in scope because it does not explicitly address linking evidence to the systems of care.

Applying the best care to a system is an extension of the precepts and foundations of EBP. Consider for a moment the evidence-based improvement equation introduced in Chapter 1 (Figure 1-3, page 15) and Figure 2-2, above.[8] Generalizable scientific evidence is at the forefront of this equation and forms the foundation of improvement. Strong experimental design and sound data analysis are vitally important to build new, generalizable scientific knowledge. Equally important is applying that evidence to a system of care and understanding the local context of care. We may make the assumption that creating the right evidence will lead to improved patient outcomes; however, the transfer of knowledge from scientific evidence to practice and improved outcomes does not occur just from the strength of evidence. So *finding* the right evidence and *applying* that evidence in practice are two separate steps. We need changes in systems of care to apply evidence consistently and dependably. The Colorado model in Figure 2-1 (page 27) shows the clinical environment in which care is provided (which includes organizational support, mentoring, facilitation, and leadership) to be an important contextual factor in the use of evidence. We'll cover context and systems of care in Chapter 4. This chapter focuses on finding the right evidence to improve systems.

# Formulating the Right Questions

Finding the right evidence to make systems improvements begins with asking the right questions.[9] When we need to find evidence for an individual patient—such as a patient with CAP—the task is relatively straightforward. When a patient has a clinical condition and some diagnostic or therapeutic approach is not clear, we should review and appraise the evidence to guide the clinical decision making. (Of course, skills in finding and appraising evidence must be part of the repertoire.) Asking the right questions for system-level improvement is a little bit different from asking questions for individual patient care.

## Types of Questions

Questions to find evidence fall into several categories. We might ask a question that looks for a definitive answer (for example, "What are the most common causes of pressure ulcers in a patient diagnosed with spinal cord injury?"). Alternatively, we might ask a question using less definitive information (for example, "Why did this patient with a spinal cord injury develop a sacral pressure ulcer at this point in time?"). In the former case, the answer will be a specific list of the most common causes of pressure ulcers in patients with spinal cord injuries. In the latter, the answer will provide a range of options, but the clinician(s) can only surmise why the pressure ulcer occurred at this time. Similarly, we might ask specific knowledge-based questions to find evidence, such as, "What are the specific criteria for adjusting vancomycin dosing based on blood levels?" These types of questions are "background questions" and are asked most commonly by individuals without much clinical experience (see Figure 2-3, below). Background questions help to fill the gaps in one's knowledge base.[9]

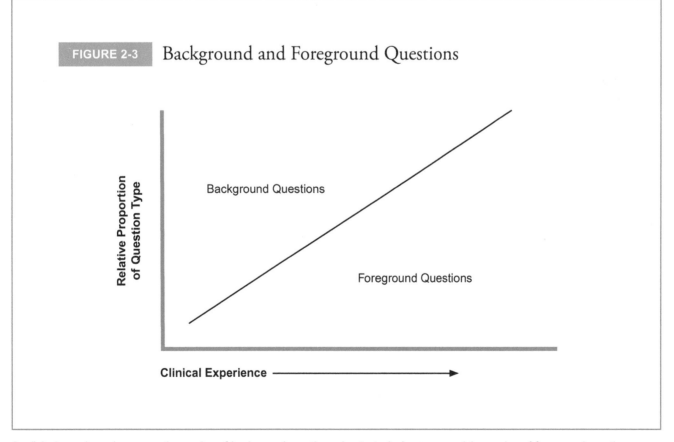

**FIGURE 2-3**  Background and Foreground Questions

Background Questions

Foreground Questions

Relative Proportion of Question Type

Clinical Experience ⟶

As clinical experience increases, the number of background questions about a topic decreases and the number of foreground questions increases. Experience is a necessary component of asking foreground questions.

## The PICO method

As experience increases, the types of questions we ask change accordingly. Foreground questions, which are more patient-centered,[9] develop. The PICO method (short for patient, intervention, comparison, outcome) helps ensure that a question is patient-centered and specific[9]:

- **Patient, Problem, Population:** Ask a question that has a definite focus for a specific patient, problem, or population. For example, "In this 82-year-old man with severe diastolic dysfunction of his heart. . . ."
- **Intervention:** Describe the diagnostic test, therapy, or prognostic factor that we need to know more about, such as "angiotensin-converting enzyme (ACE) inhibitor medicine for diastolic dysfunction."
- **Comparison:** Determine what standard to compare to either the patient or the intervention, such as, "How do ACE inhibitors compare to angiotensin II receptor blockers (ARBs)?"
- **Outcome:** Specify the clinical or diagnostic outcome to evaluate, such as "symptom relief in patients with diastolic dysfunction and monitoring of potential adverse effects."

Putting this all together, we create a comprehensive foreground of clinical questions that we can use to find evidence:

> *In an 82-year-old man with severe cardiac diastolic dysfunction, what is the efficacy of symptom reduction and potential side effects when using an ARB versus an ACE inhibitor?*

The background question about diagnostic criteria for diastolic dysfunction seeks a specific answer, while the foreground question delves more deeply into relative strengths and weaknesses of certain medications. You can see that both types of questions are important and that each has a role when looking for evidence.

## Questions to Find Evidence on Populations and Systems

Background and foreground questions can also be used to find the best evidence for populations of patients and systems. For example, we might ask a background question such as, "What percentage of patients have diastolic dysfunction chronic heart failure?" This question inquires into the epidemiology and background information regarding diastolic dysfunction for populations with congestive heart failure. It does not, however, address the epidemiology of diastolic dysfunction within a particular

setting or context. This would require a foreground question about a specific population of patients. Using the PICO method, we may inquire, "In our population of patients (*P*) with diastolic heart failure at Lake Pines Medical Center, what antihypertensive medications (*I* and *C*) should we use to decrease their symptoms and avoid potential side effects (*O*)?" This foreground population question localizes the evidence, focusing it on knowledge of the diagnosis and treatment of the condition in a specific population.

## Filtered and Unfiltered Questions, "Right" and Best Answers

Background questions tend to be more general and knowledge-based, while foreground questions probe for information and apply it in a specific way—whether for an individual patient (an 82-year-old man with diastolic dysfunction) or for a population of patients (Lake Pines Medical Center patients with diastolic dysfunction). Foreground questions are sometimes more challenging to formulate than background questions because we need clinical experience to formulate them. Also, answers to background questions have often been filtered (that is, assessed and compiled by others[9]), and we might identify the "right" answers in textbooks or in general review articles. It is often simple to identify a list of diagnostic features or treatment options for a particular condition, and this background information is essential before we progress to the more complex foreground questions. Answers to foreground questions may not be available in the same way. The literature may not provide a definite "right" answer, but we can use it to determine the best answer to guide care at a particular time. This is where the balance of the components of EBP becomes important (*see* Figure 2-1, page 27).

As we said at the beginning of this section, forming the right questions is a key first step in finding the right evidence. Having the right questions involves knowledge of the situation, and this is true whether we are searching for information for an individual patient or looking for information to apply across a particular population. Getting the questions focused and sharp is the necessary starting point in finding the information and applying it to a specific patient care situation.

# Evaluating the Strength of Evidence

Many available resources discuss the strength of evidence. You can easily obtain them on the Web with a simple search. In this chapter, we will use the materials from the Geisel School of Medicine at Dartmouth Biomedical Libraries, Evidence-Based Medicine Teaching Resources, which are available here: https://www.dartmouth.edu/~library/biomed/guides/research/ebm-teach.html. This chapter does not provide a comprehensive evaluation of research methodology or a detailed discussion of the relative strengths and weaknesses of study design and biostatistics; however, we offer a few key points that will help you evaluate the relative strength of evidence that you find.

The pyramid diagram (*see* Figure 2-4, below) summarizes the relative strength of research evidence based on the study design or resource type.[10] The quality and strength of evidence increases from the base of the pyramid to the peak.

The lower half of the pyramid contains unfiltered information, while the upper part contains reviews and syntheses that have been filtered by others.

## Unfiltered Information

At the base of the pyramid are expert opinions, case reports, and case-controlled studies. These are usually anecdotal reports of interesting findings or a consensus statement from a panel of experts about a condition for which a higher level of evidence does not yet exist. Although these often contain detailed stories of individual cases and rich narrative information, they generally do not provide the strength of evidence required to make system-level changes. The strength and certainty of the evidence increases as the research methodology increases toward the top of the pyramid.

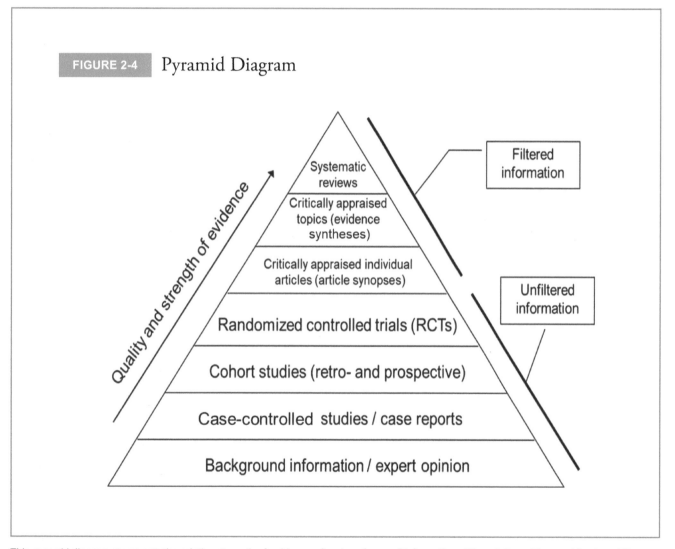

**FIGURE 2-4** Pyramid Diagram

This pyramid diagram represents the relative strength of evidence of various forms of information. Although the evidence at the top of the pyramid is considered to be the highest quality, it also has been assessed and compiled by others—that is, the information has been filtered.

**Source:** Dartmouth College. Dartmouth Biomedical Libraries: Evidence-Based Medicine (EBM) Resources. Accessed Nov 17, 2017. http://www.dartmouth.edu/~biomed/resources.htmld/guides/ebm_resources.shtml. Trustees of Dartmouth College, 2017. Used with permission.

## Cohort studies

Further up the pyramid, but still falling within unfiltered information, are cohort studies, both retrospective and prospective. Retrospective cohort studies look back at a group of individuals and determine statistically significant associations based on the data available. For example, a large database that contains information about dietary habits of individuals over several decades could be investigated to determine whether certain foods correlate with more (or fewer) heart attacks. A prospective cohort is similar, but the research questions are asked at the outset and monitored over time. These studies provide a large amount of data about each individual, and the analysis takes into account the time of the observation period—which may be many years—and the complex interaction between the factors collected. Many health services research projects that employ analysis of large databases are either prospective or retrospective cohort analyses.

## Randomized controlled trials

The final level of unfiltered information comprises randomized controlled trials (RCTs). We usually hold these as the gold standard for building scientific knowledge. RCTs build strong evidence because they control for as many factors as possible, both in the design and in the statistical analysis of these projects. Randomization—the process of assigning subjects to receive treatment A, treatment B, or no treatment at all (that is, the control group)—has the added benefit of controlling for unknown as well as known factors that might influence the outcome. The control group in an RCT provides a comparison to identify whether the changes in the intervention group are due to the intervention or due to an underlying characteristic of the group as a whole. Meta-analyses (not pictured in Figure 2-4, page 31) combine data from many studies in an effort to pool information and arrive at a conclusion.

# Filtered Information

The top part of the pyramid, above RCTs, contains sources of filtered information. These sources appraise the evidence and usually offer recommendations for practice. They may be summaries and evaluations of individual journal articles (article synopses) or syntheses of evidence from many sources (evidence syntheses). Filtered information is often convenient because someone else has gone through it and created a summary of the main findings.

## Evidence syntheses

An evidence synthesis can include evidence from a range of studies on the topic, including RCTs, cohort studies, and expert opinions. Topics can range from identification and treatment of pressure ulcers, diastolic heart failure, or even best techniques to teach patients how to use inhalers for asthma. The National Guideline Clearinghouse accessed by the medical, nursing, and pharmacy students in the opening vignette, is an example of an evidence synthesis, in which the guidelines vary in quality from those based on expert opinions to those based on higher-quality research evidence.

## Systematic reviews

At the top of the pyramid are systematic reviews, such as the Cochrane Database of Systematic Reviews. The Cochrane Collaboration is an international not-for-profit organization established in 1993 to prepare, update, and promote the accessibility of systematic reviews of the health care literature. Cochrane remains the global leader in developing and publishing evidence reviews. To date, there are thousands of reviews published online in *The Cochrane Library* in many languages (http://www.cochrane.org). Systematic reviews are generated by experts who complete structured comprehensive literature reviews, evaluate the literature, and present summaries of the findings.

## Perspectives of filtered information

When researching filtered information, it is important to understand the perspective of the authors and the sponsoring agency. For example, an evidence synthesis about CAP sponsored by an organization of infectious disease professionals may contain a focus different from that of a similar review sponsored by a home health care organization. One of them may focus on the microbiology and pharmacology for treating pneumonia, while the other may focus on nonpharmacologic interventions to help patients recuperate at home. Both foci are valid and important, but understanding the perspective from which a review is written will help you interpret the information and apply it to the clinical and improvement question.

# Level of Evidence

Identifying the level of evidence is an important step when reviewing the information. The level of evidence is a by-product of the research design. Making generalizations from case study–level data is not wise. Also, just because an article is written as a review does not mean that it contains valid conclusions or is the final word on a topic. We do not always need an extensive review of all levels of evidence for a particular condition (such as CAP). The goal is to find the best available evidence. For example, if a well-done, recent systematic review or meta-analysis is available to directly answer the clinical question at hand, then the search can end. If the systematic review is well done but not recent, we would want to look for any RCTs done since the systematic review's publication to see if there is any new evidence. If a systematic review is not available at all, then we'd look for RCTs (the study type that provides the highest-quality evidence for therapy). If we then find relevant RCTs, we could appraise them and use their evidence. If there are no RCTs, then we would look for case-controlled studies, case series, or a case study. We would search for the highest quality of evidence available to answer our particular question. The challenge is finding it.

# Choosing the Right Resource Based on the Question

The sheer number of electronic resources available can be overwhelming, particularly with their constant updates and improvements. Often we become familiar and comfortable with one or two of the most common resources. Although the specific resources may change over time, you will find it useful to be familiar with different search interfaces. Each interface has a role in finding evidence.

The Geisel School of Medicine at Dartmouth Biomedical Libraries in Hanover, New Hampshire, has a helpful guide for finding evidence-based answers to clinical questions (Table 2-1, page 34). The resources available from your local biomedical library may be similar or may be different, and resources will evolve over time.[11]

For example, when we need an overview of a particular condition (background question), print or online textbooks or summary sites are very helpful; however, summary sites likely will not contain enough detailed information if the question has a narrow focus or if we need information about a topic that was published recently. One resource, Trip Database (formerly Turning Research Into Practice), at http://www.tripdatabase.com, is freely available and searches many databases at once. The Trip database casts a wide net through evidence-based sources of systematic reviews, practice guidelines, and critically appraised topics and articles as well as MEDLINE's Clinical Queries, medical image databases, e-textbooks, and patient information leaflets. If the question encompasses a unique aspect, such as alternative therapies, or if you want to find cutting-edge information, then resources such as MEDLINE with "complementary medicine" limits for indexed journal articles or LexisNexis for news resources would provide the best options.

This list is not intended as a comprehensive compendium of every available database or search engine, but it is a reasonable starting point for finding evidence based on the need. Each of the resources listed here has strengths and limitations. Searching them on your own is a practical place to start. When you cannot find what you need, require very detailed information, or just require expert guidance, then connecting with a reference librarian is the most sensible option.

# Working with a Reference Librarian

Not too long ago—as recent as the 1990s—databases for finding evidence were not user friendly. The Internet was still in its infancy, and few institutions had high-speed Internet connections. Most libraries used a Telnet connection over traditional telephone lines that were quite slow, even for material without graphics. The interface with these tools was not a simple Web browser; rather, it required a case-sensitive and punctuation-sensitive string of characters. Reference librarians used cryptic strings of characters to retrieve evidence for clinicians and researchers. Those librarians—with master's degrees and usually on staff at biomedical libraries affiliated with health professions schools—were expert mediators for literature searches.

With the continued development of evidence search engines such as MEDLINE via Ovid, PubMed, and Google Scholar, we have entered an era of independent end-user searches. These interfaces appear simple. Many offer on-screen help and instructions, and most provide check boxes for narrowing the search criteria. The apparent simplicity in these interfaces sometimes comes at the expense of a careful, detailed search for the strongest and most reliable evidence on a topic. For a variety of reasons, ranging from a do-it-yourself mentality to embarrassment at asking for help to simply not understanding the value of librarians, most clinicians and researchers no longer enlist the help of a reference librarian.

## Levels of Literature Searches

Whether you need to use a reference librarian or not may depend on the level of your literature search. There are three broad levels of literature searches:
- **Level 1—Rapid searches:** The goal of these searches is to be quick. A rapid search is a broad stroke to capture as many resources as possible. These searches are not limited by many—if any—modifiers. For example, Google Scholar currently operates in this fashion,

**TABLE 2-1**  Finding Resources

| What Is Needed | Examples | Resources to Consider |
|---|---|---|
| **An overview of a particular disease, condition background information** | What's the difference between depression and bipolar disorder?<br><br>I have a new patient with sickle cell anemia; I need an overview of this condition. | Textbooks (print or online)<br><br>UpToDate<br><br>eMedicine |
| **Drug information** | What's the pediatric dosage of erythromycin for strep throat?<br><br>What drugs have been approved by the FDA for the treatment of Alzheimer's? | Clinical Pharmacology Online<br><br>Epocrates Online<br><br>Drug Facts and Comparisons (print)<br><br>MEDLINE for more specific information<br><br>Embase (Scopus)<br><br>ClinicalTrials.gov (registry and results database of federally and privately funded clinical trials) |
| **A synthesis of best-practice recommendations for disease management (critically appraised topics)** | What's the latest on the management of panic disorder?<br><br>What's the best method of pain control in children? | Cochrane Database<br><br>Clinical evidence<br><br>MEDLINE (Clinical Queries—Systematic Reviews category)<br><br>National Guideline Clearinghouse<br><br>MEDLINE (limit to "Practice Guidelines" publication type)<br><br>Turning Research Into Practice (Trip Database) (simultaneously searches multiple evidence-based resources) |

TABLE 2-1    Finding Resources *(continued)*

| | | |
|---|---|---|
| **An answer to a narrow question that isn't addressed in the synthesis resources (critically appraised articles and unfiltered information)** | In a 70-year-old woman with primary insomnia and a previous adverse reaction to hypnotics, can cognitive behavior therapy improve sleep quality and duration?<br><br>In a toddler with croup, does dexamethasone (or another glucocorticoid) reduce symptoms better than standard supportive care? | MEDLINE (Clinical Queries—Clinical Study Category)<br><br>ACP Journal Club<br><br>BMJ updates<br><br>Trip Database<br><br>ClinicalTrials.gov<br><br>Embase (Scopus) |
| **Evidence-based information about alternative therapies** | Is melatonin safe and effective for treating insomnia?<br><br>Does music therapy help surgical patients heal faster? | MEDLINE (limit to "Complementary Medicine" subset and "RCT" publication type)<br><br>Alternative and complementary medicine resources (for example, the Allied and Complementary Medicine Database [AMED])<br><br>Trip Database<br><br>Embase (Scopus) |
| **Cutting-edge information that isn't yet published in the journal literature (not necessarily evidence-based)** | My patient heard about a new drug on the news last night. The drug is so new that it's not in CPO or MEDLINE. Where can I find more information about it? | News resources (LexisNexis)<br><br>Web resources (Google; Google Scholar)<br><br>ClinicalTrials.gov |
| **Information to share with patients** | Where can I find some nutrition information for a patient who has been newly diagnosed with diabetes? | MedlinePlus.gov<br><br>Informed Health online<br><br>Other consumer health resources |

FDA, Federal Drug Administration; ACP, American College of Physicians; *BMJ, British Medical Journal*; RCT, randomized controlled trials; CPO, Clinical Pharmacology Online.

**Source:** Adapted from Geisel School of Medicine at Dartmouth Biomedical Libraries Web Group. Finding Evidence-Based Answers to Clinical Questions—Quickly and Effectively. Accessed Nov 17, 2017. http://www.dartmouth.edu/~biomed/resources.htmld/guides/FindingGoodAnswers.pdf.

identifying the range of resources available for a topic. The number of hits with this type of search is often quite large.

- **Level 2—Careful searches:** Careful searches often start by planning the search strategy. The searcher pays close attention to the literature types and resources that may be searched (for example, specific journals, newspaper articles, and online resources). You may start with Google Scholar but will likely need to move to a PubMed or Ovid interface to limit your search appropriately. A reference librarian is often a tremendous asset for these searches. After you find a set of resources, you can further manipulate them by limiting the set.

- **Level 3—Expert searches:** Expert searches truly demand the assistance of a reference librarian. This type of search is necessary when you need to find clinical information for a very specific question or for a rare clinical condition. Perhaps you plan on publishing a systematic review or a meta-analysis. In this case, others will scrutinize your search, so you will require expert assistance.

Reference librarians are an often-untapped source of guidance for improvement work. They are highly trained specialists who can find what you need faster and better than you can on your own. Sometimes they can even help you formulate questions. Just as improvement work on the front lines requires input from all health professionals (*see* Chapter 1), expert help can enhance your search for the best evidence for improvement.

## Summary

Because improving patient care involves closing the gap between the right care and current local performance, finding the right evidence is an important first step in improvement work. Evidence comes in many forms, and we should always search for the strongest evidence available. We need to apply EBP precepts and tools to health care systems, and not just on a patient-by-patient basis. In short, improving care for patients requires that we apply the best evidence reliably to the right patients at the right time.

## Study Questions

You are working as a student during your Obstetrics and Gynecology (Ob/Gyn) clinical rotation. The team has just completed the delivery of a 6-pound 10-ounce baby girl. Barbara Goodman, the certified nurse midwife, and you are having a cup of coffee afterward. She says, "I've heard that some are now recommending that each newborn get the first hepatitis B vaccine before going home from the hospital. This seems awfully early to start vaccines for a newborn. What have you heard in your classes?" You ponder this question as you sip your coffee, realize that you're not quite sure, so you reply, "Hmmm . . . I'm not really sure. Let me do a little looking into some evidence and see what I can find."

1. What is the appropriate background question for this clinical scenario?
2. Complete the PICO method for a foreground question:
   a. Patient, Problem, Population
   b. Intervention
   c. Comparison
   d. Outcome
3. To recommend a system-level change to the birthing pavilion at the hospital about the administration of hepatitis B vaccine for newborns, what level of evidence would you require? Why? How might you use the evidence to convince others that this is an important issue to address?
4. What resources (*see* Table 2-1, page 34) will you use to find the evidence?
5. Did you confer with a biomedical reference librarian? If so, describe what was most helpful. What might you do differently in the future in your interactions with a biomedical reference librarian?

## References

1. Agency for Healthcare Research and Quality. National Guideline Clearinghouse: Pneumonia in Adults: Diagnosis and Management. Dec 3, 2014. Accessed Nov 17, 2017. https://www.guideline.gov/summaries/summary/50009/pneumonia-in-adults-diagnosis-and-management?q=community+acquired+pneumonia.
2. Mandell LA, et al. Infectious Diseases Society of America/American Thoracic Society consensus guidelines on the management of community-acquired pneumonia in adults. *Clin Infect Dis.* 2007 Mar 1;44 Supple 2: S27–72.
3. Oxman AD, et al. Users' guides to the medical literature: I. How to get started. The Evidence-Based Working Group. *JAMA.* 1993 Nov 3;270(17):2093–2095.
4. Cullen L, et al. Sigma Theta Tau International position statement on evidence-based practice February 2007 summary. *Worldviews Evid Based Nurs.* 2008 Jun;5(2):57–59.

5. Goode CJ, et al. The Colorado Patient-Centered Interprofessional Evidence-Based Practice Model: A framework for transformation. *Worldviews Evid Based Nurs*. 2010 Dec;8(2):96–105.

6. Lewis S. Toward a general theory of indifference to research-based evidence. *J Health Serv Res Policy*. 2001 Jul;12(3):166–172.

7. Scott IA. The evolving science of translating research evidence into clinical practice. *ACP J Club*. 2007 May–Jun;146(3):A8–11.

8. Batalden PB, Davidoff F. What is "quality improvement" and how can it transform healthcare? *Qual Saf Health Care*. 2007 Feb;16(1)2–3.

9. National Association of Science Writers. How to Research the Medical Literature: Framing Specific Foreground and Background Questions in an Evidence-Based Way. Brown N. Nov 1, 2001. Accessed Nov 17, 2017. https://www.nasw.org/users/nbauman/habrown.htm.

10. Dartmouth College. Dartmouth Biomedical Libraries: Evidence-Based Medicine (EBM) Resources. Accessed Nov 17, 2017. https://www.dartmouth.edu/~biomed/resources.htmld/guides/ebm_resources.shtml.

11. Dartmouth College, Biomedical Libraries Web Group. Finding Evidence-Based Answers to Clinical Questions—Quickly and Effectively. Accessed Nov 17, 2017. http://www.dartmouth.edu/~biomed/resources.htmld/guides/FindingGoodAnswers.pdf.

# Identifying a Focus for Improvement

 ## Objectives

**After reading this chapter, you will be able to do the following:**

1. **Identify elements of a system that need to be improved, informed by knowledge of the needs of the people to be served by the system.**

2. **State ways to narrow the focus of improvement work.**

3. **Write an aim statement with a time frame for improvement that is specific, measurable, attainable, reasonable, and has a time frame (SMART).**

## Improvement Opportunity

### Primary Prevention

They are puzzled. Maria Martinez, a first-year medical resident, and Dave Thomas, a nurse practitioner student, are sitting at a conference room table with the attending physician, the nurse practitioner, and a few members of the clinic's quality improvement (QI) team. They are discussing possibilities for improving the continuity of care at the free clinic where they all work. Maria and Dave are struggling with an assignment to identify something to improve in the clinic, a requirement for their clinical rotations. They had spent considerable time thinking about several possibilities, but after presenting their ideas to the team, they felt overwhelmed. Dave looks at Phil Morrison, the attending physician, and then at the whiteboard that lists possible improvement projects. Finally, he asks, "How can we decide? There are too many things that need to be improved, and we just don't know where to start."

Phil turns to the board, reviews the list aloud, and says, "Which of these is most important to the patient population we serve: patient waiting time, evidence-based treatment of urinary tract infections, diabetes care, preventive services, or the reporting of x-ray findings to patients? We have a long list, but we need to start somewhere." Aaliyah Simpson, the nurse practitioner, speaks up, "Let's look at our data and then ask ourselves, "Which is most important to the health of our patients? What concerns us the most? What are our patients and families concerned about?"

Maria and Dave look again at the quality data from the clinic and realize there are big gaps in primary prevention. They know this is an important aspect to the free clinic population, as these interventions prevent disease from ever starting. In the first six months of her residency training, Maria tried to use a template for preventive care, but this approach left her frustrated. Dave is concerned about the lack of time available to address preventive care during a scheduled visit. He suggests that a team approach consistent with a patient medical home model may be the answer. Maria and Dave look at each other and nod. Dave turns to

the group and says, "We'd really like to improve disease prevention for patients in our clinic." Aaliyah replies, "Great! Identifying something in our system that needs to be improved is the first step. The next steps are to focus that idea and then to create an aim statement. We can discuss ways to focus your idea when we meet again later this week."

An integral component of improving health care is to focus or narrow the improvement efforts. The Model for Improvement (*see* Figure 3-1, right)[1] is a useful guide to ensure success of these efforts. This chapter addresses the first question in the figure: "What are we trying to accomplish?" To answer this question, it is helpful to go through a three-step process:

1. Identify a general area to improve.
2. Narrow the focus.
3. Create a global aim statement to guide the project.

## Step 1: Identifying an Improvement Area

So how do you find potential areas to improve? One way is to start by looking at the systems you are a part of. As you will learn in Chapter 4, a system is a set of interdependent elements working together to achieve a common aim. These elements may be both human and nonhuman (for example, technology, equipment, information). Even as a student, you are a part of many systems: a personal system with a pattern of eating, sleeping, exercising, and studying; an educational system of clinical groups, lab groups, and study groups; and clinical care systems, such as those in a nursing clinical rotation or a medical clerkship. In each of these systems, you interact with various people, processes, and structures. The goal is to create clinical systems in which all the elements (people, processes, structures) work together to achieve care that is safe, effective, patient-centered, timely, efficient, and equitable.[2]

As a student, you will certainly see opportunities for improving processes in the clinical system. Learners' unique perspectives can add to clinical improvement efforts. For example, medical students studying patient safety events as part of a clinical clerkship proposed changes that were more

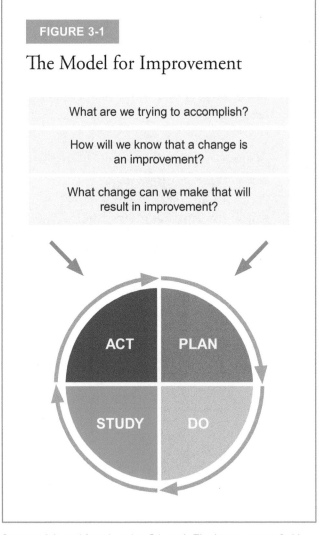

**Source:** Adapted from Langley GJ, et al. *The Improvement Guide: A Practical Approach to Enhancing Organizational Performance,* 2nd ed. San Francisco: Jossey-Bass, 2009. Printed with permission.

robust than those suggested by professionals reporting similar issues.[3] And one fourth-year nursing student, in his clinical rotation on an orthopedic floor, found that care was not always consistent with the evidence-based practice of turning patients every two hours to prevent pressure ulcers. The nursing student knew this was important both clinically and financially, as hospitals would no longer be reimbursed for any hospital-acquired pressure ulcers. Anywhere systems and processes exist, they can be improved, and identifying opportunities to improve is an important first step.

Identifying improvement areas in clinical care requires that you reflect on the care delivered, viewing it through an "improvement lens" of mindfulness (being aware of how your practice is affecting the patient) and systems thinking (looking beyond what you do and considering all the factors that affect the quality of your patient care). By definition, systems thinking links a person's behavior to the environment. In the delivery of health care, this involves understanding and valuing how the components of the complex health care system influence the care of an individual patient.[4] We can apply systems thinking throughout the continuum of care, from the individual to the health system overall. Figure 3-2, below, shows an example of care approaches that represent different levels of systems thinking.

## Approaches to Identifying Improvement Areas

The following approaches will help you identify an improvement area at the system level:

- **Seek out the patient's perspective.** Opportunities for improvement must be informed by knowledge of the needs of the people served. Review formal patient feedback results. Identify some areas you are curious about. Learn more by talking directly with a few patients about their experiences.
- **Examine point-of-care issues.** At the system level, think about what you see in practice. Do you see any procedures that do not follow policy? Are there gaps between evidence-based practice and what you see happening every day?
- **Think about the quality of care delivered.** Are there gaps in quality, as defined by the Institute of Medicine: safe, effective, patient-centered, timely, efficient, and equitable?[2]
- **Review unit- or system-level data.** Almost all clinical units will have data about the quality of care delivered. In the acute care setting, for instance, unit- and health system–level data are available for issues such as pressure ulcers, falls, infections, and readmission rates. How do those results compare to national benchmarks?
- **Discuss and reflect on frustrations.** Still another way that ideas for improvement may arise is from discussions with colleagues and organizational leaders about their frustrations with the system. Frequently all you need to do is ask, "What is the one process that frustrates us the most?" Often your frustrations reflect gaps in meeting the needs of the patients you serve.

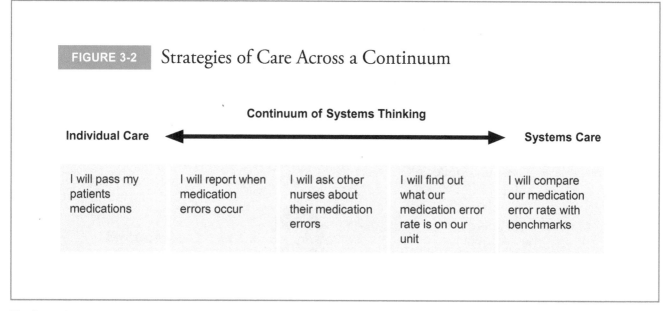

**FIGURE 3-2**  Strategies of Care Across a Continuum

Continuum of Systems Thinking

Individual Care ⟵⟶ Systems Care

| I will pass my patients medications | I will report when medication errors occur | I will ask other nurses about their medication errors | I will find out what our medication error rate is on our unit | I will compare our medication error rate with benchmarks |

The figure above illustrates multiple levels of systems thinking.

**Source:** Dolansky MA, Moore SM. Quality and Safety Education for Nurses (QSEN): The key is systems thinking. *Online J Issues Nurs.* 2013 Sep 30;18(3):1. Printed with permission conveyed through Copyright Clearance Center, Inc.

- **Seek out the perspective of the institution's leaders.** Understanding the priorities of the institution often leads to partnership with key personnel and resources.

These approaches likely will produce many potential improvement ideas. It is important to prioritize the list you generate by considering the population served, best practices, and the greatest patient needs. After you have identified the general area in which you would like to make improvements (for example, ensuring evidence-based treatment of urinary tract infection), the second step is to narrow the focus.

# Step 2: Narrowing the Focus of the Improvement Work

*Dave and Maria, the nurse practitioner student and the first-year medical resident, mull over this question: "Given what we've learned about how our clinic is doing, what is most frustrating to us about preventive care here?" They are aware that the care in the free clinic is a team effort that includes the patient and many professionals: administrative assistants, medical assistants, nurses, and clinical provider colleagues (that is, other resident physicians, nurse practitioners, and attending physicians). Maria and Dave have a conversation in the hallway with Nick Borysenko, a medical assistant. The three of them briefly review the work of all the team members. As the medical assistant, Nick obtains the chief complaint, triages the urgency of the visit, and takes the vital signs. As a nurse practitioner student and medical resident, Dave and Maria each have a primary care panel. Together, the three colleagues examine the data and find that only 10%–22% of their patients are receiving counseling on healthy living. They are frustrated about the difficulty in providing healthy living guidance to patients. In the limited time allotted for appointments, there are important prevention topics—such as diet modification, exercise counseling, and tobacco avoidance—that they often are not able to cover in any great depth.*

*Nick shares Dave and Maria's passion to provide counseling on healthy living for all the patients in the clinic. In the team meeting later, everyone agrees that this would be an appropriate goal for an improvement project; diet and exercise counseling do not get enough emphasis in care providers' time with patients. Phil, who also works as an attending physician in other clinics, says to the group, "Hmm. That's helpful to hear that you all find this to be an issue.*

*Tell me about the template for healthy living that you currently use. How much information is on it?"*

*Maria tells the group about the three main parts of her evidence-based preventive medicine template: (1) guidelines for preventive treatments such as vaccinations; (2) screening information for services such as mammograms and colonoscopies; and (3) healthy living counseling, including diet and exercise guidance. Nick points out that healthy living counseling is the responsibility of the clinic's providers and that the preventive guidelines and screening are standardized for the whole clinic. Dave has his own healthy living counseling approach, which he developed in his previous work as a clinic nurse. Nick states, "Almost all the providers have a healthy living counseling approach . . . and they're all different."*

*Dave sums it up: "All right, so this is simple. Our focus will be to 'implement an evidence-based preventive medicine template for the patients at the medical center clinic.'"* *Aaliyah, looking thoughtful, says, "Well . . . we're getting closer. You've done a great job of narrowing the focus. When we meet next, let's address the third step—that is, to craft a clear global aim that will guide the entire project."*

As we saw in the opening vignette, Dave Thomas and Maria Martinez are frustrated with the range and number of opportunities that they see need improvement in the clinic. Like many professionals, they find it difficult to narrow what they want to improve and feel overwhelmed by wanting to address everything. It's important to narrow the focus. For example, an improvement team in a primary care practice might begin with the goal of improving care for patients with diabetes, including glycemic control, hypertension and lifestyle changes. Although each of these is worthy of the team's attention, creating an improvement project that is too broad is a common pitfall. A team that doesn't appropriately narrow the focus of its goals may endure many iterations and travel several paths without achieving real improvement in any area. This leads to wandering work, unclear priorities, and frustration.

**❝❞ A team that doesn't appropriately narrow the focus of its goals may endure many iterations and travel several paths without achieving real improvement in any area.**

## Criteria to Focus Improvement Work

If you've done research, you've learned how important it is to narrow the focus of a research question. Hulley and colleagues describe a strong research question as having five characteristics: *feasible, interesting, novel, ethical,* and *relevant (FINER).*[5] We can use these criteria to focus improvement goals. Although research and QI are different in implementation and execution, they both share the common goal of generating new information; both are potential opportunities for students to publish with their mentors. Here we use the FINER characteristics as a way to narrow the focus of QI work.

*Feasible.* Your improvement project should be *feasible* within the practical limits of your situation. A project that you work on as a student team might be very different from a project you would lead as an attending physician or a registered nurse. The feasibility of the project must match with your current position and authority to act within your professional discipline.

*Interesting.* The topic for an improvement project should be *interesting* to you and to your organization. Look for a project that you are passionate about and is of interest to the stakeholders whose collaboration (including resources) you will need. For instance, a medical resident worked with a nurse QI expert to lead a project developing and testing a protocol that identified low-risk patients presenting to the emergency department with chest pain. Based on the literature, they were able to select patients for whom rapid follow-up with an outpatient workup was appropriate. Through their work, 1,735 patients had their chest pain rapidly and safely evaluated without the discomfort of hospitalization, for an estimated savings of more than $16 million in professional and facility charges. A project born of the passion of a resident interested in cardiology won the support of patients, physicians, health system leaders, and insurers.[6]

*Novel.* An improvement project should be *novel.* In Chapter 1, we discussed the fact that improvement work is the act of implementing the best practice in a local setting. Improvement work generally does not generate new, generalizable knowledge in the same way that research does, but it provides an opportunity to learn about local systems and make changes that are important to the people served by those systems. Improvement work will generate new local knowledge about a system, and it allows you to optimize the performance and outcomes of local processes, whether the project involves improving preceptorships for

fourth-year nursing students or increasing the use of appropriate antibiotics for patients with pneumonia.

*Ethical.* Your improvement project should be *ethical.* This is an essential up-front consideration when choosing a project. There should be assurances that the project poses no threat of physical or psychological harm to individuals and that there will be no invasion of privacy. It is important to have early consultation with local improvement project sponsors and the Institutional Review Board (IRB) to determine whether IRB review is required. An IRB is a committee designated to approve, monitor, and review research to protect the rights and welfare of research subjects, and this committee has the authority to determine whether QI work should be considered research. IRB practices may differ somewhat from institution to institution. A thorough review by the Hastings Center in 2006 showed that most institutional IRBs at that time were ill prepared to evaluate improvement projects.[7] Since that report was published, IRBs have instituted policies to examine the ethical issues surrounding QI projects. Although improvement work and research share many characteristics, improvement of care is integral to the delivery of care; therefore, the protection of patients during improvement activities should be part of a transformed system of accountability in clinical care. Be sure to consult with professionals who have improvement experience to help guide the team through the local improvement process, including when to involve the local IRB. Remember that the IRB itself is the ultimate decision maker about ethical oversight. Maintain a low threshold for asking their opinion. Ogrinc and colleagues published an instrument (reproduced in Figure 3-3 on page 45) to help clinicians differentiate between clinical research and QI.[8] More information about distinguishing between QI and clinical research with human subjects can be found in Chapter 9.

*Relevant.* An improvement project needs to be relevant. For clinical improvement projects, it is important that the topic be relevant to patients, staff, and administration. For example, the Veterans Health Administration (VHA), a component of the US Department of Veterans Affairs (VA), commenced a large improvement effort across 40 institutions to reduce falls and injuries due to falls in hospitalized patients.[9] The VHA—both nationally and also from local VA hospitals—committed funding, personnel, and support for the improvement work. Patient falls are high-profile events for patients and families, and injuries from falls (such as hip fractures or head injuries) can add increased length of stay and costs to a patient's

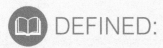

hospitalization.[10] This issue was of high importance to the patients, to the individual VA hospitals, and to the national VA. Each facility identified a passionate, interprofessional work group that consisted of physicians, nurses, physical therapists, and occupational therapists. This example demonstrates how a focus of improvement (reducing falls and injury due to falls) is relevant for all stakeholders in the organization—patients, families, clinicians, administrators—at both local and national levels. Tight alignment of priorities—those of patients, providers, hospitals, and the national VA—was an important element for keeping this project relevant and reducing falls.

## Step 3: Creating a Global Aim Statement

After narrowing the focus of the improvement work, your third step is to create a global aim statement. Starting improvement work without a clear global aim statement is akin to conducting research without a clear hypothesis. Absence of clear direction often leads to wasted time and effort. A clear aim will keep a project on track, help identify the process, and aid in identifying proper measures. Now that we have discussed some of the characteristics of finding

a project and narrowing the focus, we'll try to put it all together by developing a global aim statement. Let us return to our scenario to discover what a clear global aim for a project looks like.

*The improvement team agrees that a project focused on implementing an evidence-based template for preventive care is doable and would be of interest to many in primary care. Although the project might not be particularly novel, it would serve an important patient need and might be very useful for other clinics. Dave and Maria meet with the chair of the IRB. Together they review pertinent ethical considerations and discuss if they should request a formal IRB review. The chair informs Dave and Maria that because this is clearly about implementing best practice and not testing a new intervention, it is QI work and would not require an IRB review.*

*Later, Maria opens the team's discussion on how to focus the project: "So we started with this goal: 'Improve the healthy living counseling for the patients at the free clinic.' Then we narrowed the goal to implementing an evidence-based template for preventive care. This is a reasonable start, but the aim statement should be more specific. Will we implement the template for all patients in the clinic?" Nick replies, "It would be quite a feat to work with all the patients! We have at least a dozen providers, nurses, and administrative assistants. Perhaps our first efforts should involve only a few practitioners."*

*Dave agrees: "Perhaps we could start with something like this: 'Over the next six months, we will implement an evidence-based prevention template for three providers' patients in the clinic.'" Refining the aim helped the group feel as if it has a clear direction.*

As our scenario continues to unfold, we see how the team develops a global aim from an initial general goal to improve preventive care, dig deeper into the issues surrounding the delivery of preventive care, evaluate the feasibility and relevance of the project, and create a clear and concise global aim statement. The team is now positioned to use its aim statement as a guide for analyzing the process of care (described in Chapter 4), developing measures (described in Chapter 5), and identifying interventions to test change (discussed in Chapter 7) in the clinic system. See Sidebar 3-1, page 46, to read more about the relationship between setting aims and achieving excellence.

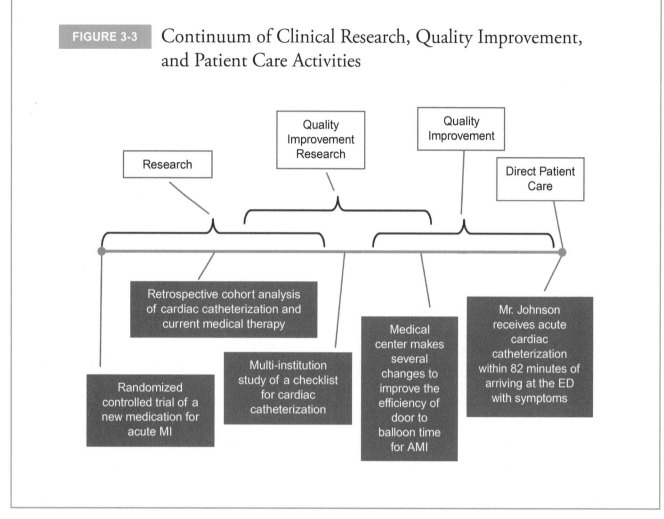

Clinicians can use this instrument to differentiate between clinical research and quality improvement. MI, myocardial infarction; AMI, acute myocardial infarction; ED, emergency department.

**Source:** Ogrinc G, et al. An instrument to differentiate between clinical research and quality improvement. *IRB: Ethics & Human Research.* 2013 Sep–Oct;35(5):1–8. Printed with permission from Copyright Clearance Center, Inc.

## Using SMART Criteria to Define a Clear Global Aim Statement

In many ways, the global aim statement for an improvement project reads like the first sentence of a newspaper article. In one sentence of a newspaper article, you know *what* happened *where, who* was involved, *when* it occurred, and perhaps even *how* it transpired. The aim for improvement work should be equally descriptive.

Components of an effective aim statement can be described with the SMART criteria.[11] The first criterion is that an aim needs to be *specific* (S) and can be sharpened by including the who, what, where, when, and why components. Next, an aim needs to be *measurable* (M) and include concrete

criteria for assessing progress toward attainment of the goal. The aim should also be *attainable* (A) and *reasonable* (R), and it must represent an objective that is achievable and that you are willing and able to work toward. Finally, an aim needs to be grounded within a *time frame* (T).

Here is an example to illustrate the components of a SMART aim. A group of nursing students on a clinical rotation observed that the date of intravenous (IV) tubing initiation was not being marked. They knew that tubing needed to be changed every three days, per hospital protocol. Because the tubing was not marked with a date of initiation, the students were unsure when to change the tubing. They formed a QI team with the staff on the unit and proposed this aim statement: "By the end of our

Pushing System Performance to the
Theoretical Limit

Setting the goal in an aim statement almost always involves a numeric goal, such as
"25% increase in X," "decrease Y by 50%," or "improve the rate of Z from 62% to 85%."
Targets such as these are very helpful. These types of targets provide clear goals for a team;
however, why aim for only a 25% change? Why settle for 85% when you can strive to meet
100%? Providing the right care to the right patient at the right time should be the target.
When we set a goal to reach the absolute best result, we refer to it as the *theoretical limit of
performance*. In contrast, when we set a goal to meet a reachable aim, we call it an
*incremental limit of performance*.

The theoretical limit is defined as the performance of a system that is *possible*. *Possible* is
the key consideration and differs from *probable*. The probable performance, stated as an
incremental limit, is the likely level of performance that has been reported by others, perhaps
in a journal article, as a best practice at a conference, or through benchmarking. We reach
the theoretical limit by asking, "What if we were able to achieve 100% performance?" or "How
could we achieve a 0% error rate?" This can be a powerful frame of mind to push system
performance to higher levels. Sometimes the incremental limit is the appropriate goal;
sometimes the theoretical limit is the appropriate goal. The decision likely will depend on the
particular situation and the improvement team's judgment about what will be most meaningful
and motivating for the people working in the system.

A theoretical limit used as a part of a local campaign can be very motivating to staff. An
example might be "Let's reduce our sepsis rates to zero." In other situations, it may be more
realistic and achievable if the team uses an incremental limit that can be increased over time
so that staff can reach achievable goals. Sometimes teams are not satisfied with incremental
improvement (although perhaps they started with incremental goals), and they push systems
to higher performance, driven to zero—the absolute best. Irrespective of what limit is chosen,
the goal is to improve quality and safety, and the choice is somewhat arbitrary since there is
no evidence that one is superior to the other.

clinical rotation, 100% of the IV tubing will be marked
with the date that the tubing was initiated and changed."
This aim statement follows the SMART criteria: specific
(IV tubing will be marked with start and changed dates),
measurable (100% marked tubing), attainable, reasonable,
and has a time frame (by the end of the clinical rotation).

To differentiate what is a clear aim, we provide examples in
Table 3-1 (page 47) of aims developed by teams working to

decrease falls and injuries due to falls. The first example
provided is not a strong aim. The team certainly gets credit
for being honest, but the locus of control is outside the
team ("clinical manager"), and the goal is not very clear.
The second example is slightly better because it contains a
defined location ("2-South") as well as a time frame ("one
week"); however, the goal is not clearly defined, and the
time frame is not reasonable.

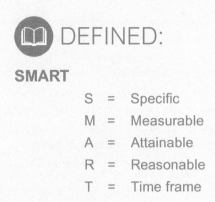

The third example is an aim that is specific and concise and meets the SMART criteria. It gives the specifics of the project (exactly who will be working on this project and where they will focus), the desired measurable outcome ("reduce by 25%"), and a time frame to guide the project ("over the next six months"). The aim also is attainable and reasonable as stated. A stated time frame is an important element when chartering a QI project. Stating a time frame gives a clear message to all involved that this is not a team that will stagnate but one that will reevaluate its goals at reasonable intervals. This final example will serve the team well as it starts making changes on 2-South. It will help to refocus the team as data roll in and the team evaluates whether any of the changes have led to improvements in care. Clear aim statements are vital for the success of any improvement project, whether it is a personal project, an educational project, or a clinical project. In Chapter 7 the global aim statement is the foundation for testing specific changes, often with a series of trials (or Plan–Do–Study–Act cycles), each with its own specific aim.

## Summary

Determining an area for improvement work is not always simple. Although there are many opportunities in health care to do improvement work, we must always be mindful of the needs of the people we serve. The three steps discussed in this chapter—identifying an improvement opportunity, narrowing the focus, and creating a clear and focused (SMART) global aim statement—provide a framework to help us answer the first question in the Model

| TABLE 3-1 | Examples of Aim Statements for Reducing Falls in Hospitalized Patients |
|---|---|

| Sample Aim | Characteristics |
|---|---|
| **Unclear Aim:**<br>Our clinical manager directed us to reduce falls in patients. | • Identifies main purpose<br>• Has a locus of incentive that is external to the team<br>• Does not include a time frame or a measurable goal |
| **Unclear Aim:**<br>On Ward 2-South, we will reduce patient falls over the next week. | • Contains clear description of the location of the improvement work<br>• Does not include a measurable goal or a description of the team<br>• Has a time frame that is not reasonable or attainable |
| **Clear Aim:**<br>Working with the falls reduction team on Ward 2-South, we will reduce the rate of patient falls by 25% over the next six months. | • Is a very clear aim that meets SMART criteria (specific, measurable, attainable, reasonable, and has a time frame) |

for Improvement: "What are we trying to accomplish?" Creating a clear and focused global aim statement during the planning of an improvement project will save time and energy downstream and will keep the project focused as it moves forward. The aim statement serves as a summary of and a compass for the project.

# Study Questions

## Identifying Opportunities for Improvement

Each of the following scenarios describes either an educational or a clinical situation in need of improvement. There may be several aspects of the situation that require improvement. After you read each scenario, determine where you might focus your improvement efforts and describe your reasoning.

### Scenario 1

As you complete your first six months as a medical student at your preceptor's office, you reflect on what a wonderful experience it has been. You get plenty of time to see patients on your own, and your preceptor even observes some part of your interview and/or examination at every session. You have been fully integrated into the practice, and sometimes you even arrive early on your preceptor day to attend the lunchtime practice meeting. It seems like a good way to grab a bite to eat and learn about how this small, rural practice operates.

At this month's practice meeting, the office secretary is concerned about a recent decrease in the availability of urgent care appointments. The nurse states that several appointments per week are available for women who complain of pain and burning with urination. Your preceptor explains that these visits are necessary to evaluate the possibility of a kidney infection and to determine the proper antibiotic regimen for the suspected urinary tract infection. You recall reading an article about using a nurse triage protocol on the phone to treat simple urinary tract infections. Your preceptor asks for your input on how to address this problem.

• What can you suggest to get this started? Why would you suggest this plan? What would be your aim?

### Scenario 2

You are a nursing student doing a clinical rotation on a general medical floor. Your patient is a 60-year-old male with type 2 diabetes admitted for the third time this year with hyperglycemia. The physician is frustrated because he has been working very hard to improve this patient's glycemic control. The patient continues to be in poor control; his most recent hemoglobin A1c was 9.3% (normal is less than 6%). You talk with the patient, and you find that he is overwhelmed by having to make so many lifestyle changes. You decide to use your improvement skills and develop with the patient an aim statement using the SMART criteria. The patient shares that he mostly struggles with doing finger sticks at home.

• What would the aim statement be in this scenario?

## Identifying and Evaluating the Components of an Aim Statement

For each of the following clinical improvement scenarios, indicate whether the aim statement is consistent with the SMART criteria (specific, measurable, attainable, reasonable, has a time frame). If it does not meet one or more of these, then state how the aim could be improved to include more or all of the criteria.

### Scenario 1

Gosia Nichols is a third-year medical resident in obstetrics and gynecology. Many patients who are only a few weeks pregnant will present to the clinic with vaginal bleeding. This is commonly termed a miscarriage, or an incomplete spontaneous abortion. Although this is a relatively common presenting condition, Gosia has been frustrated. She has recognized that the treatment that is recommended for this condition depends on who is the attending in the clinic that day. Some attending physicians prefer medical management, some prefer surgical management, and some prefer watchful waiting. Gosia uses her elective in practice-based learning and improvement to develop a plan to address this issue. After reviewing the literature and identifying the evidence-based guidelines for treatment of incomplete spontaneous abortions, she prepares an aim statement for her work:

*Aim:* Over the next 24 months, we will increase the use of evidence-based treatment by 25% for first-trimester incomplete spontaneous abortions at the residents' clinic.

• Write an improved aim statement for this scenario.

### Scenario 2

Throughout his first year in nursing school, Fadi Mathias has been frustrated by the students' use of information technology. He worked for an Internet company before coming to nursing school and knows that wikis, listserves, and blogs could help the students communicate more effectively. Currently, most of the students (as well as faculty and administration) use only e-mail to communicate. Fadi would like to develop a free online community for his classmates, but he is not sure which online tools would be used the most. He teams up with several other students and a faculty leader, and they chart a course to address this issue.

*Aim:* Through the use of focus groups and a survey, identify and implement online community tools for first-year students.

- Write an improved aim statement for this scenario.

## Scenario 3

Since John Fariq began medical school, he has wanted to complete a residency in orthopedic surgery. Now that he has the opportunity to do a sub-internship, John is very excited to make a good impression. Although he enjoys the excitement of the operating room, he finds evaluating patients in the orthopedic clinic less interesting. Through the first 10 days of this rotation, he is particularly bothered by how often the x-rays are not available for the team in the clinic. This creates delays and frustrations for the patients and the staff as the right information (x-ray) is not available to make decisions for patients. Sometimes when an x-ray cannot be retrieved, the patient is sent for a repeat x-ray film. This wastes time for everyone. John decides to help solve this problem and presents an aim statement to his faculty preceptor.

Aim: Working with the orthopedic clinic staff, we will decrease the rate of missing x-rays by 50% over the next three weeks.

- Write an improved aim statement for this scenario.

# Analyzing Ethical Considerations of Improvement Work

For each of the following scenarios, describe the ethical challenge that should be addressed.

## Scenario 1

Ed Stepstein was excited to be working on a project to improve the safety of unfractionated heparin use in the intensive care unit (ICU). As a fourth-year nursing student,

he had some experience with the considerable variability in the partial thromboplastin times (PTTs) of patients treated with unfractionated heparin. His QI elective was an opportunity to work with a team in the ICU to show how few patients had therapeutic PTTs. Ed spent several hours at one of the computer workstations at the hospital, reviewing charts and lab results. He created a comprehensive database that listed the patients, the dates of admission, and the PTT lab values for all patients treated with unfractionated heparin in the past 12 months. He was eager to begin the analysis, so he copied the file to his thumb drive and headed home to continue his work after dinner on his home computer.

- What cause for concern does this scenario illustrate? (Answer: Patients' personal health information must be kept private. Data collected for QI must be held to the same standards of privacy as any other personal health information. Transferring data to a thumb drive and to a personal computer puts these data at risk. The data should either be stored on a secure server at the hospital or should be de-identified.)

## Scenario 2

Ana Zamar is excited about being a first-year internal medicine resident and developing her own patient panel. She enjoys the relationship building and physician–patient interactions that occur over time. She feels fortunate to have attended a medical school that emphasizes practice-based learning and improvement and systems-based practice, and she believes she is ready to build and improve care for her patients. Having just heard about a new diabetes medication that was recently released, Ana writes a clear aim (with the SMART criteria to guide her work). She sets up a small electronic database of her patients who have diabetes and sends out a letter to every other patient on the list, informing them that they will be starting on this new medication. She is excited to track the results and see if the new medication improves diabetes outcomes for her patients.

- What cause for concern does this scenario illustrate? (Answer: This is closer to a research project than a QI project. Assigning a new drug to half the patients without tailoring the treatment is not applying best evidence to patients. There are many choices for diabetes medications, and those treatment options need to be chosen for each individual patient. Also, Ana is testing a new medication in a group of patients without first obtaining their consent to do so.)

# References

1. Langley GJ, et al. *The Improvement Guide: A Practical Approach to Enhancing Organizational Performance,* 2nd ed. San Francisco: Jossey-Bass, 2009.

2. Institute of Medicine. *Crossing the Quality Chasm: A New Health System for the 21st Century.* Washington, DC: National Academy Press, 2001.

3. Hall LW, et al. Effectiveness of patient safety training in equipping medical students to recognise safety hazards and propose robust interventions. *Qual Saf Health Care.* 2010 Feb;19(1):3–8.

4. Dolansky MA, Moore SM. Quality and Safety Education for Nurses (QSEN): The key is systems thinking. *Online J Issues Nurs.* 2013 Sep 30;18(3):1.

5. Hulley SB, et al. Designing Clinical Research, 4th ed. Philadelphia: Lippincott Williams & Wilkins, 2013.

6. Adeola O, et al. Patients identified as low risk may be safely discharged from the emergency department after presentation with chest pain. Abstract presented at the American Heart Association Scientific Sessions, Orlando, FL, Nov 2015.

7. Baily MA, et al. The ethics of using QI methods to improve health care quality and safety. *Hastings Cent Rep.* 2006 Jul–Aug;36(4):S1–40.

8. Ogrinc G, et al. An instrument to differentiate between clinical research and quality improvement. *IRB: Ethics & Human Research.* 2013 Sep–Oct;35(5):1–8.

9. Mills PD, et al. Reducing falls and fall-related injuries in the VA system. *Journal of Health Care Safety Quarterly.* 2003;1:25–33.

10. Oliver D, et al. Risk factors and risk assessment tools for falls in hospital in-patients: A systematic review. *Age Ageing.* 2004 Mar;33(2):122–130.

11. Doran GT. There's a S.M.A.R.T. way to write management's goals and objectives. *Manage Rev.* 1981 Nov;70(11):35–36.

# Process Literacy and Systems in Health Care

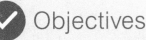 Objectives

**After reading this chapter, you will be able to do the following:**

1. **Recognize the importance of describing the process of care that is being studied.**

2. **Select from a variety of methods, including brainstorming, cause-and-effect diagrams, flow diagrams, deployment flowcharts, and work flow diagrams, to create a model to describe clinical processes.**

3. **Identify how the process of care is related to the context of care.**

 Improvement Opportunity

## Clinic Visits

"Big changes are planned." That's the buzz in the clinic as nurse practitioner Selena Delacruz and physician James Simon arrive to cover their shifts in the drop-in clinic. The drop-in clinic is the place for acute medical needs at the medical center—a step below the emergency department in patient acuity. No appointments are necessary; the clinic gives a patient the opportunity to show up and be evaluated for any general medical concern. Selena and James discover that the drop-in clinic is going to switch from being a "no appointment necessary" clinic to being an "appointments only" clinic based on concerns voiced by patients and families and the results of patient experience surveys. "This should be interesting," they both muse.

James settles in for what's sure to be a long afternoon. He looks at the pile of patient face sheets. As each patient arrives at the clinic, he or she is checked in and triaged by a nurse before his or her chart is placed at the bottom of the stack. Clinicians then pull a sheet from the top of the stack to see patients in the order in which they arrived. James has been working at the clinic for six months and has never thought this system worked well, but the process was already in place when he started there. He needs to be at the clinic only a half day per week, and he finds it easiest to go with the current flow. Selena, however, was one of the developers of the current process (which was thought to be highly innovative at the time). She is skeptical about the proposed change and thinks it may not have been properly planned.

Changes will be coming, however. The department formed a committee that recommended that all patients have appointments in order to be seen in this clinic. No one is quite sure how the new process will operate. James is not even sure how the current process is operating; he wonders whether the new process will replace the current one or serve as an alternative to it. Selena is really comfortable with the current system, although she acknowledges that it has drawbacks at times. As James and Selena grab their first charts for the afternoon, each notices the huge crowd of patients in the waiting room. They see that the front-desk workers are scrambling to get patients checked in. And in the triage room, the nurses are busy assessing the severity of each patient's chief complaint. As they take all this in, James and Selena wonder just how well the patients' acute care needs are being met here at the medical center.

# Process Analysis

A *process* is a series of actions or procedures that result in some outcome. Processes are inherent in our daily lives. For example, waking and preparing for work or school consist of a series of actions such as showering and eating breakfast that result in getting to work or school, hopefully on time. Health care is made up of many processes, including scheduling, triaging, and examining patients, as in the case described above. Processes in health care are not inherently good or bad, but each has developed for a reason. Sometimes a process develops because it is the most efficient way to provide care to patients; sometimes processes develop because of patient or family feedback; some processes exist because they are convenient for billing purposes; and some processes help an organization comply with rules and regulations.

Although all members of the health care team are part of many activities, they are often process illiterate. *Process illiteracy* is a lack of familiarity with what actually happens, day-to-day, from other points of view such as from the patient and family or from other members of the health care team. Perhaps even more concerning is *process arrogance*—an exaggerated sense of knowing how things work. Many feel that they know processes because they work in the environment. But health care is complex. Process arrogance is usually not a deliberate decision, but rather it is a sense that develops over time due to exposure to routines. Because health care processes tend to be complex interactions among clinicians, administrators, patients, families, information, and technology, no one person can fully experience health care processes from all vantage points. Knowing structures, patterns, and people within an organization leads to *process literacy* and is a vital step in the improvement of systems.

## The Importance of Process Analysis

Knowing a process and how it operates is important for improving care. Process analysis—including the measurement of key steps of the process—is crucial to improvement for three reasons.

*Process analysis provides a common picture—a shared model—for an improvement team.* Each member of the team experiences the work flow differently. The administrative staff, the front-desk staff, nurses, physicians, medical assistants, and the pharmacist all have information about what actually occurs. Describing the process of care from the patient's and family's point of view with input from all the stakeholders—including patients and families—creates a shared visual model that everyone can use and understand. This model is an important tool for keeping the patient experience at the center of the conversation about improvement.

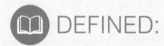 DEFINED:

**Process**
*Process* is a series of actions that result in some outcome.

**Process Illiteracy**
*Process illiteracy* is a lack of familiarity with what actually happens, day-to-day, from other points of view.

**Process Arrogance**
*Process arrogance* is an exaggerated sense of knowing how things work.

*Process analysis helps identify which parts of the system are important to measure in order to understand and improve the care system.* When a team studies a process, the team can identify several different measures to improve it. For example, a team working to improve care for patients with myocardial infarctions may consider measuring pain management in the emergency room, the percentage of patients who receive beta-blockers, and the percentage of patients who receive coronary angioplasty with stenting of coronary vessels. They may also consider patient satisfaction, the number of days a patient misses work, the experience of the family of an acute myocardial infarction patient, or the number of patients who proceed to coronary artery bypass graft. These are all important considerations, but a team cannot measure and monitor all of them at the same time in a focused improvement project. Process analysis helps a team identify and prioritize the measures through the identification of key leverage points. (Chapter 5 describes the identification and linking of measures to a process.)

*Process analysis helps generate hypotheses for change* (Chapter 7). When a team starts its work to improve something, many team participants will think they know how to make the process better. These individuals may be on the right track, but creating a visual model of the process will generate a greater number of possible improvement approaches. This work helps a team see redundancy and waste in the system and figure out where the team might rearrange or combine steps in the process. Similar to doing a history and physical on a patient before creating a list of possible diagnoses, process analysis collects data that will generate ideas and lead to improvement.

Understanding the process is the first step in generating a visual representation of the process, sometimes called a *process model.* A process model is akin to creating a surgical plan for a patient. Surgery is much more than cutting, suturing, and tying knots. Successful surgery involves several steps, such as preparing the surgical site, assessing the patient's level of anesthesia, assessing the surgical site, accessing the anatomic location, completing the surgical intervention, and closing the surgical site. Each of these steps contains many subprocesses that the surgical team performs. For example, because of the complex steps involved in a surgical procedure, it is vital that the care team understand both the anatomy and the physiology of the patient, each of which will affect the surgical approach. Similarly, process analysis identifies the anatomy of a system (in our case, a part of a health care system). It determines the approach to improvement and makes improvement efforts more successful. In a careful and thoughtful process

analysis, improvement team members can share their knowledge of a system of care, build a common understanding of how the system works, identify measures, and create a list of possible changes.

# Process Analysis Methods

There are many ways to analyze a process. We will explore a few of the methods that are available to study any process. Depending on the size and scope of an improvement project and the process to be understood, one or more methods are often used in combination. Becoming familiar with the methods discussed here (as well as other methods) provides a range of options to describe and understand processes of care. We present several of these tools, identify their strengths and limitations, and explore an example of each related to this chapter's opening vignette (*see* Table 4-1, page 54).

## Brainstorming

Brainstorming is a common tool used by groups to create a large list of ideas in a short time. This technique allows all team members to get involved in problem solving and can provide input to other process analysis tools. A common method for brainstorming is to have all members of the team write down their thoughts about the process on a sticky note and then share with the group without judgment about the value of their ideas. When brainstorming is appropriately facilitated, it can lead to a range of ideas that provide important insights into the processes of care. Table 4-2 on page 55 shows the results of the opening vignette team's brainstorming session, demonstrates how this works. Having several people in the system of care involved in brainstorming helps the team identify aspects of the process that may have been hidden. For example, the front-desk check-in clerk on the improvement team described her challenges with the drop-in clinic. Although the drop-in system is also frustrating for the nurses and physicians, clinical staff are physically shielded from the waiting area. The front-desk clerks bear the brunt of patient inquiries. When patients become frustrated or angry with a long wait time, the front-desk clerks are left to manage the problems. The brainstorming session helped everyone involved to realize that this process encompasses more than just the clinical staff. The clinic support staff are key to the process as well. Any solutions for improvement will need to take this into account.

## Cause-and-Effect Diagrams

A cause-and-effect diagram (also called an Ishikawa, or fishbone, diagram) is an excellent tool for uncovering and

| TABLE 4-1 | Strengths and Limitations of Basic Process Modeling Techniques[1] | |
|---|---|---|
| **Modeling Technique** | **Strengths** | **Limitations** |
| **Brainstorming** | • Enlists input from many individuals<br>• Can be an important starting point<br>• Generates a wide range of ideas and possibilities<br>• Helps build a sense of ownership in the improvement work | • Brainstorming in a group must be facilitated.<br>• Must move beyond generating possibilities<br>• Be wary of getting "stuck" on barriers. |
| **Cause-and-effect diagram** | • Standard way to identify barriers in a system<br>• Clearly identifies the end product of the system in the "head"<br>• Stems and leaves identify specific aspects of the process. | • No time aspect to the diagram (cross-sectional analysis tool)<br>• Might be limited by the domains on the stems |
| **Flow diagram** | • Shows the parts of the process<br>• The diagram is based on the entire process, not a standard template, so all the steps in the process are shown.<br>• Standard symbols make interpretation easier.<br>• Can be annotated | • No clear link to individual or professional responsibilities<br>• May become long and too detailed<br>• Can become cluttered by annotations |
| **Deployment flowchart** | • Same symbols as standard flow diagram<br>• Shows people who perform each step<br>• Columns for measures and change opportunities | • Challenging to fit on one sheet of paper<br>• Often difficult to represent complex process with many stakeholders |
| **Work flow diagram** | • Uses a diagram of the physical layout to map the work flow pattern<br>• Can show flow of people, information, or materials<br>• Can often identify areas of duplication, waste, and handoffs in a process | • Challenging to show multiple patterns or variations in flow<br>• Need accurate depiction of the physical layout of an area<br>• Nonstandard processes might not show a consistent pattern. |

**Reference**

1. George ML, et al. *The Lean Six Sigma Pocket Toolbook: A Quick Reference Guide to Nearly 100 Tools for Improving Process Quality, Speed, and Complexity.* New York: McGraw-Hill, 2005.

**TABLE 4-2** Summary of Brainstorming Session by Drop-in Clinic Improvement Team (Nurse Practitioner, Physician, Front-Desk Clerk, Physician Assistant, and Patients)

| Discussion Question | Summary of Discussion |
| --- | --- |
| What works well at the current drop-in clinic? | • Each patient is seen on the day of his or her choice.<br>• Not having to make appointments enables patients to simply show up at the clinic.<br>• Other services in the hospital can refer patients to the clinic for evaluations.<br>• Medical and nursing students get exposure to a range of urgent care conditions.<br>• If the patient volume is low, the clinic's work may be completed early in the day. |
| What can be improved at the drop-in clinic? | • Although they do not have the information, front-desk clerks are often forced to field questions from patients about when they might be seen.<br>• Patients do not know when they will be seen by a clinician.<br>• Patient volume and acuity are difficult to anticipate.<br>• If the patient volume is high, the clinic can run several hours over the limit.<br>• Staff (clerks, nurses, clinicians) feel that they have very little control over the patient flow in the clinic. |
| How do we want to provide acute care for our patients? | • Our patients need access to acute medical care at our medical center.<br>• The staff in the acute care area should have control over the flow in the clinic and be able to match available staff with patient volume. |

describing the range of factors that influence an outcome. There are three steps to creating this type of diagram:

1. A cause-and-effect diagram starts with the empty template (*see* Figure 4-1a, page 56). The box at the right side of the diagram contains a statement of the current problem to be solved. This is the effect, or the outcome, of the process being studied. This statement should be concise and to the point. This is not the same as the aim statement (Chapter 3) of the improvement team but just a clear statement of the specific problem. In Figure 4-1a, the statement is "Patients, staff, and clinicians are frustrated by long wait times in drop-in clinic."

2. The next step is to create headers (broad categories) for the stems on the diagram. Traditionally, six headers can be used: people, processes, policy, methods, materials,

and environmental factors. You may choose to use all or some of these, or you may choose to create labels that are appropriate for your team. It is prudent to use at least three headers for a cause-and-effect diagram; using more than six headers often makes the diagram cluttered (*see* Figure 4-1b, page 57).

3. The third step is to investigate each of the headers for more concrete examples. Under "People" in Figure 4-1c on page 58, for example, you can see that the team entered the comment "Many new clinicians who are not familiar with the system," indicating that the group felt that the new clinicians were having difficulty with the clinic system. There are other examples under the other domains in Figure 4-1c. Note that sometimes you may be able to use results of your brainstorming to help fill in the concrete examples under each category.

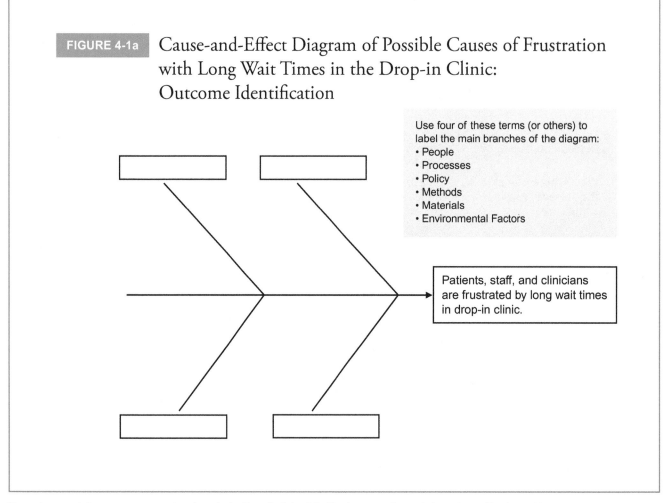

Cause-and-Effect Diagram of Possible Causes of Frustration with Long Wait Times in the Drop-in Clinic: Outcome Identification

Use four of these terms (or others) to label the main branches of the diagram:
• People
• Processes
• Policy
• Methods
• Materials
• Environmental Factors

Patients, staff, and clinicians are frustrated by long wait times in drop-in clinic.

The outcome of the current system is written in the "head" of the fish. The items on the main branches will refer to this outcome.

This process continues around the entire diagram, with specific ideas placed on each of the bones. The cause-and-effect diagram is a hypothesis-generating tool, so any reasonable contribution should be added.

## Flowcharts

A flowchart diagram uses a standard set of symbols to provide a visual image of a process that allows for study, annotation, adjustment, and ultimately agreement. An oval is the start or end of the process, a rectangle is a step in the process, a diamond is a decision point in the process, and arrows depict the flow. For example, Figure 4-2 on page 59 shows a flowchart for a patient in the drop-in clinic, the scenario presented at the beginning of this chapter. The example in Figure 4-2 shows that a large portion of the patient's time is spent in the waiting room. This validates the results of the brainstorming session: When patients become frustrated about long wait times, they approach the front-desk staff first with questions because they are the ones in close proximity to the waiting room. A standard flowchart is limited because there are no clear links to individual or professional responsibilities. Also, because it may contain many annotations, a flowchart can become quite cluttered and perhaps not easily interpreted.

## Deployment Flowcharts

Another process modeling tool, a deployment flowchart (also called a swim-lane diagram), uses the same symbols as a standard flowchart and has the added benefit of identifying the specific process steps for different team members who interact with the patient at certain stages. In Figure 4-3 on page 60, the parts of the process completed by each team member (nurse, check-in clerk, and clinician) are depicted in separate columns. A deployment flowchart can also include columns for measures of each stage of the process and opportunities for improvement at each stage of

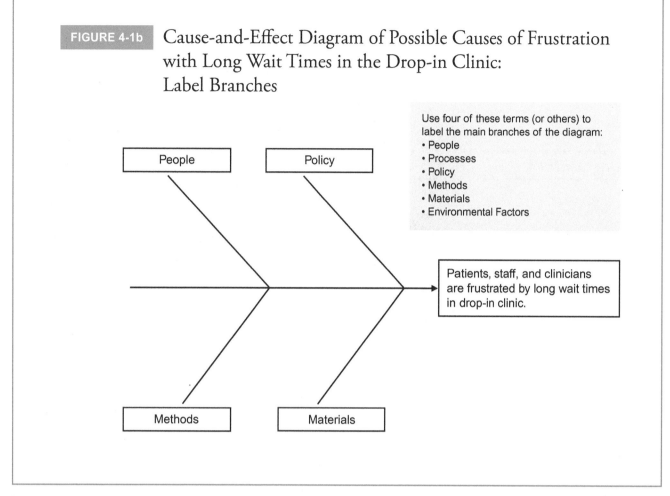

FIGURE 4-1b Cause-and-Effect Diagram of Possible Causes of Frustration with Long Wait Times in the Drop-in Clinic: Label Branches

Use four of these terms (or others) to label the main branches of the diagram:
• People
• Processes
• Policy
• Methods
• Materials
• Environmental Factors

People

Policy

Patients, staff, and clinicians are frustrated by long wait times in drop-in clinic.

Methods

Materials

Next, label the main branches with domain headers that are appropriate for the system you are evaluating. In this example, the drop-in clinic team chose People, Policy, Methods, and Materials. You may choose more than four main branches and may choose other domain headers than those suggested here.

the process. Figure 4-3 represents the same process as in Figure 4-2. You will note in Figure 4-3 that even though the patient identifies his or her visit as being with the clinician, the majority of the patient's time is spent interacting with other individuals. This demonstrates the complexity in making changes even within one drop-in clinic. The change from a "no appointment necessary" to an "appointment only" clinic will affect all who work in this clinic.

## Work Flow Diagrams

A work flow diagram (also referred to as a transportation or spaghetti diagram) uses the physical layout of a setting to show the flow of people, materials, or information. This type of diagram is effective for showing waste in movement by individuals, showing delays in processing information, and identifying places where handoffs between individuals occur.[1] Figure 4-4 on page 61 shows a work flow diagram

for one of the triage nurses in the drop-in clinic for the care of one patient. Notice how the nurse must travel from the triage room to the area by the front-desk clerk to retrieve paper from the printer, then to call the patient from the waiting room, and to another area to converse with the physician in the examination room and assist the patient to the procedure room. The movement of the nurse shows several areas of redundancy in which his or her actions could be more efficient. The work flow diagram provides a complementary process analysis to the other models when the goal is to create efficient and reliable flow in a system.

Notice how each process model (Figures 4-1, 4-2, 4-3, and 4-4) indicates that each patient spends a good deal of time waiting, but each depicts this slightly differently. There is no right or wrong process model; you can choose the one that best represents the system, context, and culture on

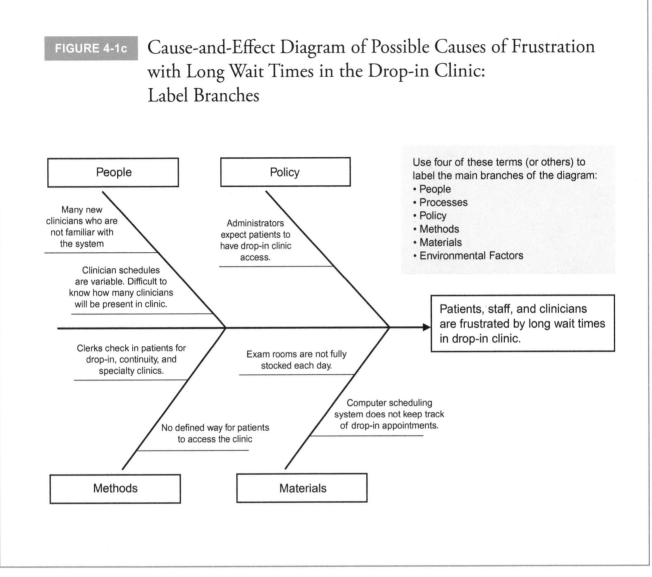

**FIGURE 4-1c** Cause-and-Effect Diagram of Possible Causes of Frustration with Long Wait Times in the Drop-in Clinic: Label Branches

People

Many new clinicians who are not familiar with the system

Clinician schedules are variable. Difficult to know how many clinicians will be present in clinic.

Policy

Administrators expect patients to have drop-in clinic access.

Use four of these terms (or others) to label the main branches of the diagram:
• People
• Processes
• Policy
• Methods
• Materials
• Environmental Factors

Patients, staff, and clinicians are frustrated by long wait times in drop-in clinic.

Clerks check in patients for drop-in, continuity, and specialty clinics.

Exam rooms are not fully stocked each day.

No defined way for patients to access the clinic

Computer scheduling system does not keep track of drop-in appointments.

Methods

Materials

Now add specific examples on the main branches. These are not to identify blame for the outcome but are to represent the range and depth of factors that contribute to the outcome.

which you are working. Sometimes, as in our example, you may even create several versions of the same process and choose the ones that are most helpful to your improvement team. With any process model, it is important to elicit feedback from everyone who is part of the process as part of the validation. Each process model the team creates should be circulated to others who are part of the process, posted in a common area with an invitation to add comments, and ideally shared with patients and their families. This vetting step will improve the process model and focus the work on what will best improve the process for patients and staff.

❝❞ There is no right or wrong process model; you can choose the one that best represents the system, context, and culture on which you are working.

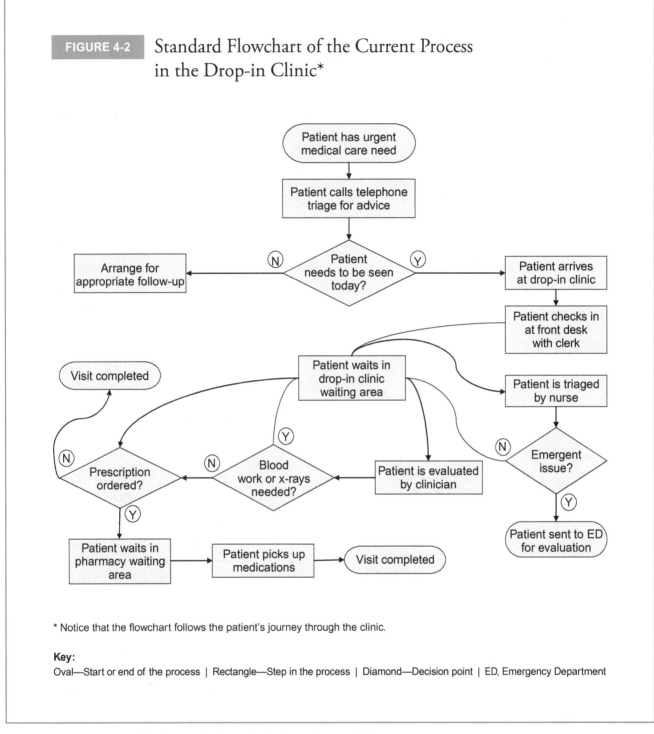

* Notice that the flowchart follows the patient's journey through the clinic.

**Key:**
Oval—Start or end of the process  |  Rectangle—Step in the process  |  Diamond—Decision point  |  ED, Emergency Department

Additional guidance on creating a flowchart is located in the Appendix, page 159.

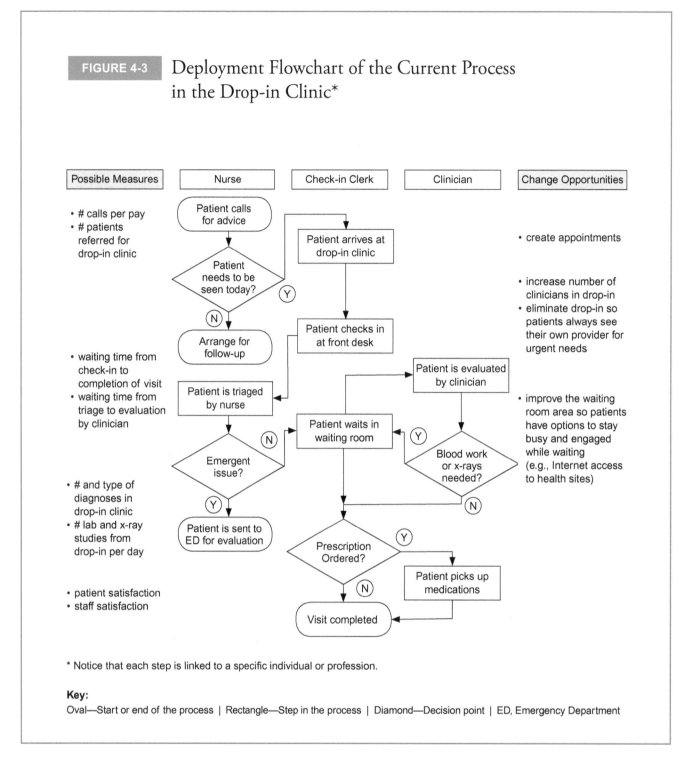

**FIGURE 4-3** Deployment Flowchart of the Current Process in the Drop-in Clinic*

| Possible Measures | Nurse | Check-in Clerk | Clinician | Change Opportunities |

- # calls per pay
- # patients referred for drop-in clinic

Patient calls for advice

Patient needs to be seen today?

Arrange for follow-up

Patient arrives at drop-in clinic

Patient checks in at front desk

Patient is evaluated by clinician

- create appointments

- increase number of clinicians in drop-in
- eliminate drop-in so patients always see their own provider for urgent needs

- waiting time from check-in to completion of visit
- waiting time from triage to evaluation by clinician

Patient is triaged by nurse

Patient waits in waiting room

Emergent issue?

Blood work or x-rays needed?

- improve the waiting room area so patients have options to stay busy and engaged while waiting (e.g., Internet access to health sites)

- # and type of diagnoses in drop-in clinic
- # lab and x-ray studies from drop-in per day

Patient is sent to ED for evaluation

Prescription Ordered?

Patient picks up medications

- patient satisfaction
- staff satisfaction

Visit completed

\* Notice that each step is linked to a specific individual or profession.

**Key:**
Oval—Start or end of the process | Rectangle—Step in the process | Diamond—Decision point | ED, Emergency Department

This diagram represents the same process shown in Figure 4-2 but has a different format.

# Culture, Context, and Systems

We indicated that the process model should reflect the culture, context, and systems in which the work is done. A process in health care is intimately related to the culture of

a clinical setting, the context of clinical care, and the health care system. We will discuss each in more detail below.

## Culture

Culture has been defined in many different ways. In a general sense, culture is used to denote a historically

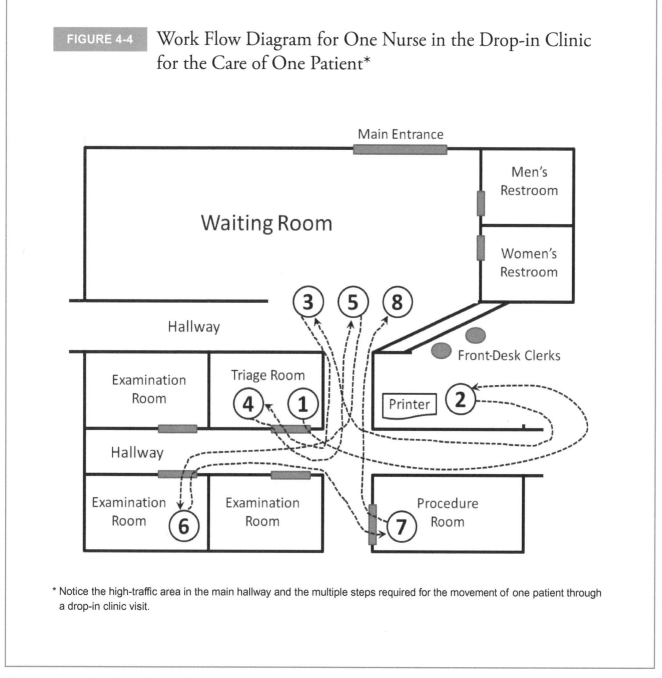

**FIGURE 4-4** Work Flow Diagram for One Nurse in the Drop-in Clinic for the Care of One Patient*

Main Entrance

Men's Restroom

Women's Restroom

Waiting Room

③ ⑤ ⑧

Hallway

Front-Desk Clerks

Examination Room

Triage Room

④ ①

Printer ②

Hallway

Examination Room ⑥

Examination Room

Procedure Room ⑦

\* Notice the high-traffic area in the main hallway and the multiple steps required for the movement of one patient through a drop-in clinic visit.

This diagram uses the physical layout of a setting to show the flow of people, materials, or information.

transmitted pattern of meanings and symbols by which people communicate and develop their knowledge and attitudes about life.[2] This definition reflects the social aspect and development of culture. *Culture* also refers to a pattern of learned, group-related perceptions—including both verbal and nonverbal language—that is added to values, the belief system, and the disbelief system.[3] This definition is important because in it, culture tells you what is true and what is not true about the system in which you work.

Students learn through this type of culture early in their clinical rotations, when more senior students pull them aside and tell them, "You learned quite a bit in your classroom work, but let me tell you how it *really* works around here."

Understanding the culture is important because it is a powerful, latent, and often unconscious set of forces that determines both individual and collective behavior. In other

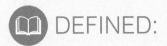

# DEFINED:

### Culture

*Culture* also refers to a pattern of learned, group-related perceptions—including both verbal and nonverbal language—that is added to values, the belief system, and the disbelief system.

words, culture has a strong influence on how both individuals and groups perform and behave and should not be ignored. It is important to understand the role culture plays in an organization when you set out to make the organization more efficient and effective.[4]

Culture is a deep, broad, and stable feature of an organization. The depth of organizational culture provides direction and meaning to an individual's work. It provides tacit rules on how to do things. Deciphering and understanding the culture of an organization takes time and provides explanations of why certain processes exist. One important feature of culture is that its stability makes it predictable. Although the predictability of work routines is often valuable, attempts to change culture often produce anxiety for everyone in the organization. The stability of culture also means that changing culture requires tackling some of the most stable (and possibly recalcitrant) parts of the organization.

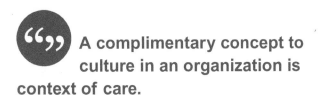

A complimentary concept to culture in an organization is context of care.

## Context

Culture is generally an accumulation over time of the actions, reactions, and artifacts within an organization. A complimentary concept to culture in an organization is *context of care*. *Context* refers to the conditions in which a particular event or situation occurs.[5] Just as context is important for understanding a story in literature, the context of clinical care processes provides a framework. Context is a local occurrence at a particular place and point

in time and is more dynamic than the culture, which is the underlying and more stable part of the organization. Common contextual elements include the practice type, patient population, geographic location, leadership structure, model of care, and technology use. It also includes less tangible elements such as behaviors and attitudes (for example, patient and staff engagement and motivation to change).[6] Context is more than just a list of elements; it is the interrelationships between these elements and how the elements and the relationships change over time.

An example of contextual differences is the supposedly similar inpatient medical units within a hospital setting. On both units, the average experience level of the registered nurse is two years. The patients on both units have similar medical diagnoses. Both units follow the policies and procedures of the hospital and the medical department. However, one unit is managed by an experienced nurse leader, while the other has a new leader with less than three years of nursing experience. In addition, one unit is part of the resident teaching service, while the other unit has a hospitalist nonteaching model of care. Even if both units choose to work on the same process for improvement, the solutions may be different based on these contextual issues. For example, if the improvement requires changes to physicians' orders, it may be simpler to implement on the hospitalist unit with a limited number of physician staff versus the resident service where providers change monthly. The context and the underlying culture should not be ignored; identifying the particular elements in the context of care is an important part of improving care.

*The complex interaction of culture and context.* Although identifying an organization's culture and context might seem simple on the surface, it quickly becomes quite complex. A health care system has many connections and interactions among its multitude of stakeholders: the patients and families, the nurses, the technology and information systems, the physicians, the pharmacists, and the administrative staff. When we consider the different ways to view culture and context, these factors—and particularly the interactions between them—become numerous. The important point here is to appreciate the complexity and depth that culture and context play in the delivery of care. A specific culture and context are not inherently "good" or "bad" but must be—and can be—recognized and described. Illustrating the processes, structures, and patterns of care is immensely helpful in making changes that are important, effective, and stable.

# Systems

Culture and context exist within the different levels of a health care system. A *system* is a set of interdependent elements working together to achieve a common aim. These elements may be both human and nonhuman (for example, technology, equipment, information). Identifying the levels of the system helps us to understand the context.

*Levels of systems.* One model for representing the levels of systems in health care is shown in Figure 4-5 on page 64.[7] This target diagram shows six nested levels of health care systems. The model helps us address the question "What system is the unit of practice, intervention, and measurement that we are studying and improving?" This model of nested levels maintains the patient at the center—the appropriate focus for all improvement activities. As we move out from the center, we encounter the individual care providers and patient system, the familiar patient–clinician dyad. The microsystem is the next level and is important because it represents the transition from "one clinician to one patient" care to "many clinicians to many patients" care.[8] The microsystem is the first level of population patient care. Moving out from the microsystem is the mesosystem, which represents the connections between microsystems (such as the information technology department or division of cardiology). The next level is the macrosystem, which is the hospital or health system. The outer circle in the model represents the community, market, and social policy systems. In the model, each level of the system can influence the patient's context of care at the center—some are proximal and some are more distant from the patient and family experience.

Let's take a closer look at each level:

- **Self-care system:** The self-care system is the patient, the information, and the information technology needed to take action to maintain health or increase the level of personal well-being. For example, a patient who has asthma will take medicines daily and will monitor environmental triggers that might make the asthma worse. Perhaps she will monitor peak expiratory flow rate (PEFR) each day to track the progress of her asthma.
- **Individual care provider and patient system:** If you ask a patient, "Where do you get your health care?" the patient may respond, "I see Mary Jones, a nurse practitioner at the Pines Medical Clinic." This reflects the system level of the clinician's relationship to the patient and family as well as the aim of their interaction (control of asthma symptoms in this example). The aim of this interaction is important and differs depending on the type of practice and training of the clinician.

- **Microsystems:** Microsystems are a unique part of the health care system. They comprise the people who come together to care for a defined population of patients and their families.[9] Microsystems are clinicians, clinical and administrative support persons, information, information technology, and a defined group of patients who come together for a specific health care purpose. The technology and information transferred between individuals is also part of the microsystem. The microsystem is a rich source of the context that influences the process on the front lines of care. The patients and families are a key part of the microsystem—not only on an individual basis but also on a population basis. The microsystem is the level at which you can start to identify and make changes for groups of patients.
- **Mesosystem:** The mesosystem is the middle level of care delivery in an organization. It is the place where microsystems are linked and interact for patient care. This level is often identified by a service line (such as cardiac care center) or a department (such as medicine or nursing). Mesosystems often need to work together for a specific episode of care. For example, a patient with asthma who has an exacerbation presents to the urgent care clinic, requires admission to the intensive care unit for several days, and then completes her hospitalization on one of the medicine wards. Although she experienced care in three separate microsystems, her path through this episode was through the department of medicine mesosystem. However, systems at the same level can interact with one another. This patient could also be viewed as experiencing care in the department of nursing. This demonstrates the complexity of the systems approach to understanding care. The circles in our model do not depict the actual complexity of health care systems but provide a strong starting framework.
- **Macro-organization system:** A hospital, a clinic, or an integrated health care system that cares for a larger population is the macro-organization system. This can be either a single hospital or an integrated health network that cares for a group of patients across a region.
- **Society, community, market, and social policy system:** This is the geographic, political, and/or economic group of macro-organizations (for example, hospitals, payers, government) that have the aim of providing health care and fostering health in a community. For example, this part of the health care system encompasses the laws and regulations that influence the health care of patients. These elements generally influence the policies and health care options that are offered through insurers, hospitals, microsystems, and individual providers, but can also directly influence individual patients, as seen with health care reform changes.

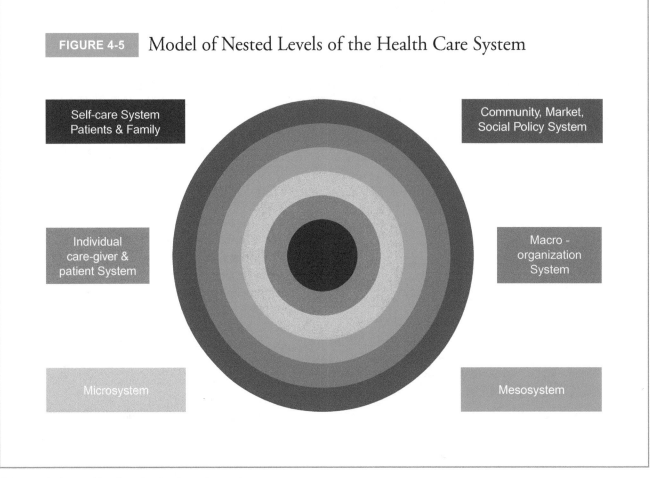

## FIGURE 4-5  Model of Nested Levels of the Health Care System

**Self-care System Patients & Family**

**Community, Market, Social Policy System**

**Individual care-giver & patient System**

**Macro-organization System**

**Microsystem**

**Mesosystem**

This model of nested levels maintains the patient at the center.

Source: Adapted from Nelson EC, Batalden PB, Godfrey MM, editors. *Quality by Design: A Clinical Microsystems Approach.* San Francisco: Jossey-Bass, 2007. Printed with permission.

*Interactions among system levels.* The model in Figure 4-5 is helpful in showing the different levels of the health care system, but how do these all fit together? Earlier, we mentioned a patient with asthma who monitors her PEFR at home. Let's suppose she has an office visit with her primary care provider every four months to review medications and symptoms (a patient–provider system). Between office visits, the patient has many interactions with the microsystem. She logs her PEFR values at a website that is reviewed regularly by a respiratory therapist affiliated with the provider's office. Also, the patient takes advantage of a home visit arranged through the local hospital (macro-organizational level). A nurse conducts the home visit to help the patient identify local environmental triggers for her asthma and to recommend changes to decrease the influence of the triggers. Although these health care workers are part of separate microsystems, they are under the

mesosystems of the departments of medicine and nursing at the hospital. Finally, the patient is influenced by social policy and the health care market. She is a member of a health insurance plan that has changed the formulary recommendations for asthma medications, so she must switch brands of inhaled corticosteroids. This brief example shows that while the patient remains at the center of the health care system, her care may be affected by the many elements that occur at all levels of the system.

Culture, context, and systems are intimately linked to the processes of care. By understanding these elements, the members of an improvement team can create a more reliable picture of what really happens for their patients. Input from all the team members helps identify the cultural and contextual elements that influence efforts to improve care.

# Summary

Process literacy is an important step in improving care. A common model of the care process is produced for the improvement team to discuss. In the Model for Improvement (*see* Figure 1-6 on page 21 in Chapter 1), a process model provides the necessary bridge between identifying measures and making changes. There are many tools available to create a process model. As with any other set of tools, practice and trial-and-error are key in helping to develop skills. You can practice developing and interpreting process maps of the processes around you such as your morning routine, your study patterns, or a patient visit at a clinical site or hospital. Creating a visual representation builds process literacy and provides insight into the many people, patterns, and structures involved in the delivery of care.

# Study Questions

The following scenario describes a clinical care process in which a woman needed a stat C-section to deliver her baby. After you read the scenario, you will complete a fishbone diagram to determine some of the causes for the delay in the process. You will then create either a process flowchart or a deployment flowchart to depict what occurred. Finally, you will review the fishbone diagram and the process map to identify opportunities to improve this process.

*Physician Magda Mooney is worried. She is driving to the hospital quickly, and her pager is ringing again. She knows that Emily LaFountaine presented to the labor and delivery ward ready to deliver. Her contractions are about 4 minutes apart, but her cervix is not expanding as quickly as would be expected. When Magda was called at home 10 minutes ago, it was obvious that the patient needed a C-section as soon as possible.*

*Magda arrives at the labor and delivery ward and is surprised to see that Emily is still in a delivery room. The charge nurse says that the hospital policy is to not move the patient to the operating room (OR) until the attending physician is present. Now Emily needs to be transferred to a gurney and transported to the OR. Oh, great—a delay. And where is the nurse anesthetist? He was supposed to arrive before the physician to place the spinal needle for anesthesia for the C-section. The labor and delivery clerk says that the call schedule had been changed at the last minute, so she had been paging the wrong on-call person. They figured out who was on call, and he is just arriving at the hospital. Another*

*delay! At least Emily looks comfortable, and the baby's vital signs are looking okay, too.*

*Finally, the OR crew is assembled, and the patient is in the OR. The team performs a successful C-section, but the first incision occurred 52 minutes after the decision was made to go to C-section. National guidelines state that the decision-to-incision time should be less than 30 minutes. The mother and the baby are doing fine, but the frustration with the stat C-section process is evident to everyone. If only they could understand some of the issues that cause such variability in this process.*

1. Complete the fishbone (cause-and-effect) diagram (*see* Figure 4-6, page 66). Start at the "head" of the fish, with a clear and concise statement of the problem. Then fill in the boxes with categories. Finally, add specific items to each of the main branches.
2. Create a process flowchart or a deployment flowchart of the current process in this scenario. Be clear about where the process starts and where it ends. You may add extra details that may not be apparent in the description of the case. Remember that you are creating the process as it exists, with all the challenges and problems, not the ideal process.
3. Generate a list of possible changes that may be tried to fix this problem. Use your fishbone diagram and flowchart to guide your decision making.

## References

1. George ML, et al. *The Lean Six Sigma Pocket Toolbook: A Quick Reference Guide to Nearly 100 Tools for Improving Process Quality, Speed, and Complexity.* New York: McGraw-Hill, 2005.
2. Geertz C. *The Interpretation of Cultures.* New York: Basic Books, 1973.
3. Singer MR. *Intercultural Communication: A Perceptual Approach.* Englewood Cliffs, NJ: Prentice-Hall, 1987.
4. Schein EH. *The Corporate Culture Survival Guide: Sense and Nonsense About Culture Change.* San Francisco: Jossey-Bass, 1999.
5. Merriam-Webster. Context. Accessed Nov 21, 2017. https://www.merriam-webster.com/dictionary/context.
6. Kaplan HC, et al. The influence of context on quality improvement success in health care: A systematic review of the literature. *Milbank Q.* 2010 Dec;88(4):500–559.

7. Nelson EC, Batalden PB, Godfrey MM, editors. *Quality by Design: A Clinical Microsystems Approach.* San Francisco: Jossey-Bass, 2007.

8. Batalden P, Ogrinc G, Batalden M. From one to many. *J Interprof Care.* 2006 Oct;20(4):549–551.

9. Nelson EC, et al. Microsystems in health care: Part 1. Learning from high-performing front-line clinical units. *Jt Comm J Qual Improv.* 2002 Sep;28(9):472–493.

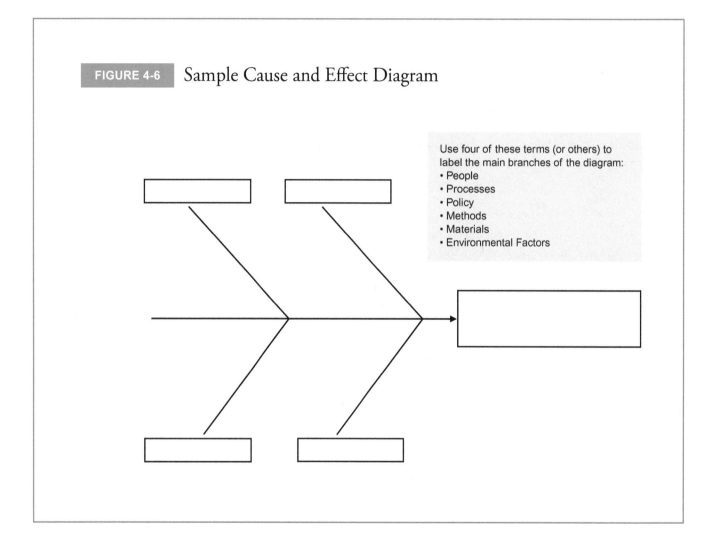

**FIGURE 4-6** Sample Cause and Effect Diagram

Use four of these terms (or others) to label the main branches of the diagram:
- People
- Processes
- Policy
- Methods
- Materials
- Environmental Factors

# Measurement Part 1: Data Analysis for Decision Making in Health Care Objectives

 ## Objectives

**After reading this chapter, you will be able to do the following:**

1. **Explain why data are necessary for the improvement of health care.**

2. **Describe the differences between data used for research, accountability, and improvement.**

3. **Define the concept of a balanced set of measures for improvement work.**

4. **Practice identifying measures for improvement.**

 ## Improvement Opportunity

### Interprofessional Team Approach

It's time for interprofessional patient rounds. Douglas Mandel, a surgical physician intern in his second month of residency training; Elizabeth Larsen, a nurse on the surgical floor with eight years of experience; Tiffany Kaliaydan, a pharmacist; and Brett McHenry, a dietitian, are all in attendance. Their first patient is Annette Quinn, a 73-year-old woman in post-op day three for a partial colectomy for her persistent bleeding and symptoms of diverticulitis. As Douglas greets her with a "Good morning," he notices that she looks concerned. She tells the team, "My belly hurts a lot this morning . . . the incision seems to be burning. It felt better yesterday." Elizabeth, the nurse, reports that the patient had a fever of 101°F (38.3°C) this morning and that the midline incision was reported as looking swollen, red, and angry. A small amount of pus was draining from the inferior part of the wound. After the team examines Annette, Douglas explains to her that it appears she has an infection and needs intravenous antibiotics.

The team finishes rounding on the other patients. Douglas approaches the attending general surgeon, Teresa Rollins, who has many years of experience with patients, surgical technique, and complications. As they discuss Mrs. Quinn's wound infection, Teresa listens to the story and comments, "That's certainly a risk with abdominal surgery. Be sure to remain sterile in the operating room and carefully change dressings post-op."

Tiffany, troubled by this reply, says, "I read an article about the appropriate timing of preoperative antibiotics. When I checked the chart, I saw that Mrs. Quinn's antibiotics were not started on time and that she received only one dose. The guidelines recommend that antibiotics be started before the incision is made and continued for 24 hours afterward.[1] It appears that Mrs. Quinn never received any antibiotics after the surgery. Do we know how often this occurs?" The attending ponders this question and replies, "I understand why those guidelines are important. Guidelines are often helpful, but they also can interfere with your decision making as a physician. Sometimes it just feels like 'cookbook medicine.' Wound infections are always a risk of surgery, particularly abdominal surgery." Douglas pushes back, "But perhaps this is an issue for other patients on the surgical service, too?"

Elizabeth returns and says, "I was able to get some data about post-op wound infection from our unit manager. We've had an 18% increase in postsurgical infections on the unit over the past eight months." The attending glances at the numbers and says, "Hmm . . . that's a cause for concern. Much higher than I would've guessed. Perhaps we should look into this in a little more detail." The rest of the team is energized by the information in the data that Elizabeth shared. They all agree to form a quality improvement (QI) team to work on this, and also invite one of the QI patient volunteers to join the team. Now they have the team to investigate and improve the timing of perioperative antibiotics. They make a plan to meet later that week to get started.

# Importance of Data for the Improvement of Health Care

Unfortunately, the attending physician's attitude in the above vignette is sometimes too common. For many years, health care workers were entrusted by the public to provide high-quality care. The public saw this as the professional duty of these workers and assumed it would occur due to the extensive schooling and training of each health care worker. The public, and more specifically patients, believed that because clinicians gained knowledge and skills from school and clinical training, they were capable of providing reliable and high-quality care. Health care professionals focused on the care of each individual patient and determined outcomes by how each patient fared. As one physician said, "There may be a 5% chance of that complication, but if it happens, it happens 100% to that patient." Health care will always focus on each individual patient, but there has been a clear shift and imperative to evaluating outcomes of groups of patients, individual providers, and groups of providers. This shift in perspective is rooted in outcomes research and data evaluation. Using data to evaluate outcomes is necessary for the improvement of health care.

## Historical Foundations for Using Data to Improve Care

The foundation for using data to understand the outcomes of medical care and offer suggestions for improvement was seen as early as the mid-1800s. Central to this development were a young army nurse and a medical student.

### Florence Nightingale's polar-area diagram

Florence Nightingale's work as a nurse for the British army is an excellent example of using data for improvement in health care. During the Crimean War (1853–1856), she traveled with the army and cared for injured soldiers in the field hospital.[2] She was appalled to find that the mortality rate for soldiers in the field hospital was much higher than for soldiers at home in England. She recognized that while many soldiers were injured, the soldiers seemed to be dying more from complications of their wounds rather than from the wounds themselves. Her first step was to notice the difference in the care and the outcomes. Within just six months of her arrival at Scutari (located in what is now Istanbul), the improvement of sanitary conditions resulted in the mortality rate's dropping from 42.7% to 2.2%. Perhaps more impressive is that she devised a way to display the data and track the progress each month. Her polar-area diagram (also called a coxcomb chart) is a combination of stacked bar and pie charts and depicted the monthly number and causes of deaths (see Figure 5-1 on page 69). Her presentation of data was so effective that *The Times of London* published the work and shared it with Parliament. Most importantly, her data display and analysis were the key to sharing the outcomes and the message with others, which led to interventions that greatly improved hospital sanitation and lowered mortality.[2]

FIGURE 5-1 Polar-Area Diagram

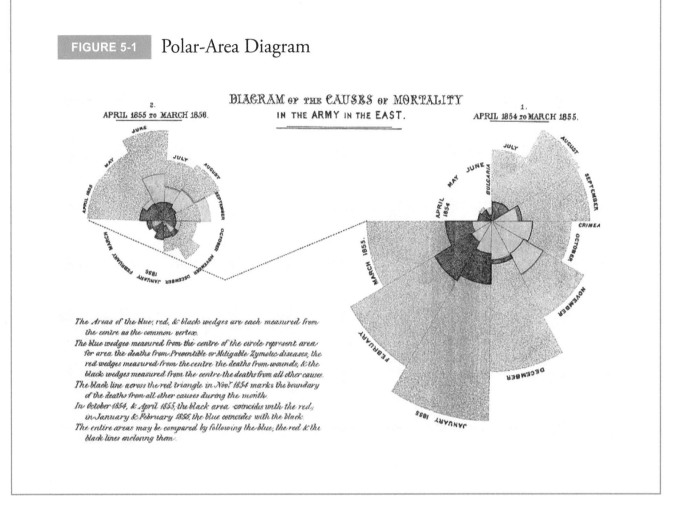

Polar-area diagram (also called a coxcomb chart) of preventable deaths of British soldiers per month during the Crimean War as analyzed by Florence Nightingale.

**Source:** Nightingale, Florence. *Notes on Matters Affecting the Health, Efficiency and Hospital Administration of the British Army.* London: Harrison & Sons, 1858.

## Ernest Codman's end result system

In the late 1800s in Boston, Ernest Amory Codman was a medical student at Harvard.[3] During his surgery rotation, the medical students were responsible for administering anesthesia. One of his colleagues, Harvey Cushing, had a patient who became nauseated, vomited, and died as a result of this nausea and vomiting. The attending surgeon shrugged off the nausea and vomiting as a usual part of anesthesia and surgery. Codman and Cushing were disappointed with this attitude and began competing to see who could have the best patient outcomes in surgery. Some of the first medical records resulted from this competition. The colleagues created anesthesia cards that tracked the patient's name, operation, attending surgeon, complications, and a graph of vital signs during the operation (*see* Figure 5-2 on page 70). These "end result"

cards were simple and straightforward, and contained just the data that Codman and Cushing were tracking for their surgical patients.

Codman was passionate about the outcomes of patient care. His *end result system* was his term for monitoring and assessing the outcomes of every patient encounter and creating a compendium of data for the patient until the end result became clear. He created the first patient registry. At a time when there was little, if any, record of patient progress or outcomes while in the hospital, Codman pushed for records of each and every patient encounter. He hoped to push medicine from "art" to "science," but this was a notion whose time had not yet arrived. When he presented his system to colleagues and hospital leaders, he was ostracized. Others did not want to know the outcomes. His passion for

**FIGURE 5-2** "End Result" Card

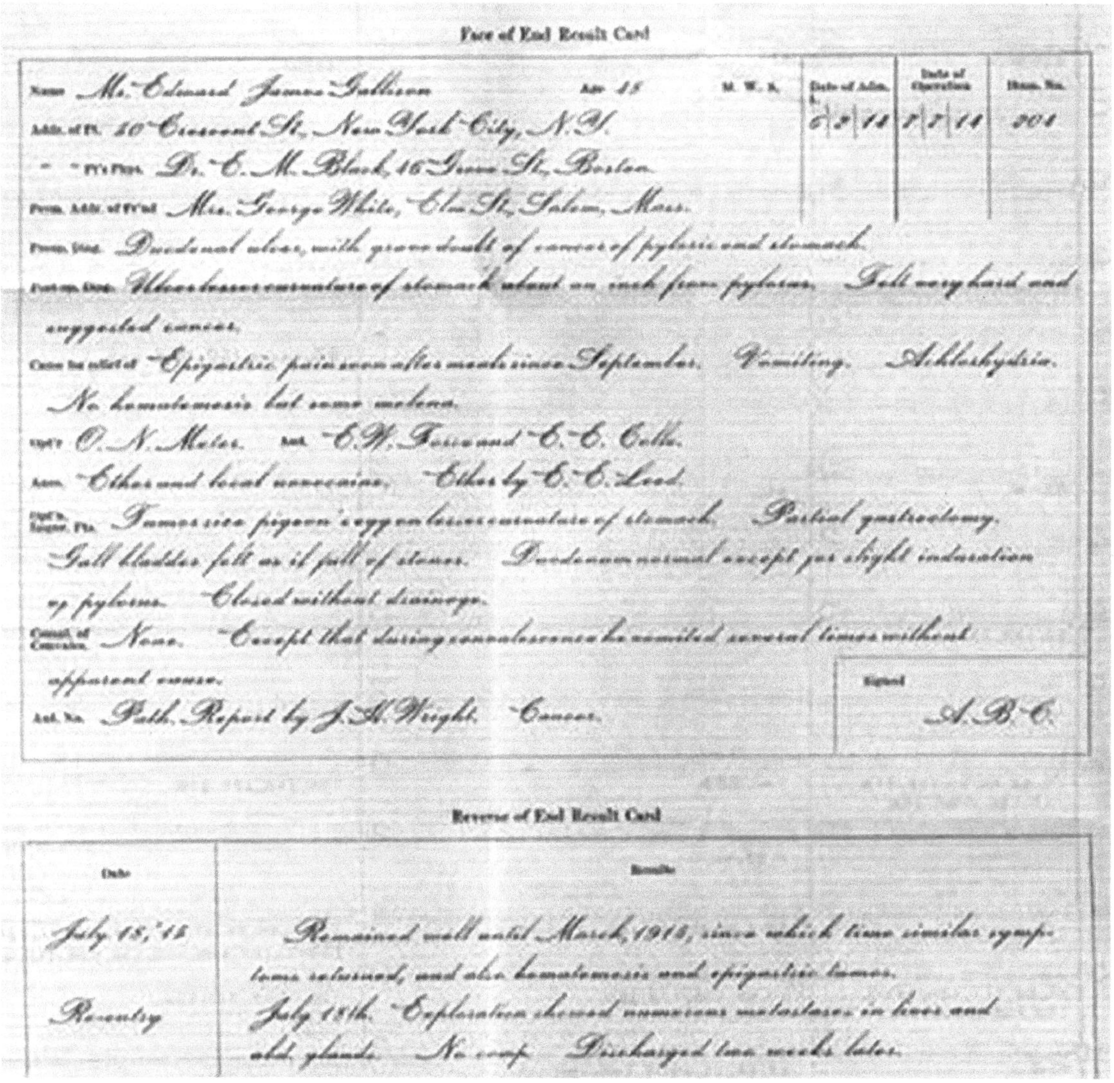

Face of End Result Card

Name Mr. Edward James Gallison Age 45 M. W. S. Date of Adm. 6/8/14 Date of Operation 8/8/14 Hosp. No. 201

Addr. of Pt. 20 Crescent St., New York City, N.Y.

" " Pt's Phys. Dr. E. M. Black, 16 Grove St., Boston

Perm. Addr. of Fr'nd Mrs. George White, Elm St., Salem, Mass.

Prem. Diag. Duodenal ulcer, with grave doubt of cancer of pylorus and stomach.

Post-op. Diag. Ulcer lesser curvature of stomach about an inch from pylorus. Felt very hard and suggested cancer.

Cause for relief of Epigastric pain soon after meals since September. Vomiting. Achlorhydria. No hematemesis but some melena.

Opr'r O. N. Meter Ast. E. W. Townsend E. C. Cotts

Ans. Ether and local novocaine. Ether by E. C. Lord

Opr'n, Surgeon, Fin. Tumor size pigeon's egg on lesser curvature of stomach. Partial gastrectomy. Gall bladder felt as if full of stones. Duodenum normal except for slight induration of pylorus. Closed without drainage.

Compl. of Convales. None. Except that during convalescence he vomited several times without apparent cause.

Aut. No. Path. Report by J. H. Wright. Cancer.

Signed A. B. C.

Reverse of End Result Card

| Date | Results |
|---|---|
| July 18, '15 | Remained well until March, 1915, since which time similar symptoms returned, and also hematemesis and epigastric tumor. |
| Recently | July 18th. Exploration showed numerous metastases in liver and abd. glands. No comp. Discharged two weeks later. |

Example of anesthesia "end result" used by Avery Codman (© 1910). Notice the simplicity of the information: patient name, age, gender, medications administered.

**Source:** Codman EA, *A Study in Hospital Efficiency; As Demonstrated by the Case Report of the First Five Years of a Private Hospital*, Boston: [privately published], 1917.

the end result system resulted in a loss of income and stature in the medical community; however, his system was groundbreaking and served as the foundation for medical records that are used by health care professionals today to establish accountability, monitor quality, advance clinical science, allocate resources, and even stimulate informed choices by patients and physicians.

## Continued Struggles in Applying Data to Improve Care

Nightingale and Codman collected and analyzed data to understand the system of care. Their most significant contributions, however, were not the mere act of collecting data and detecting patterns but rather that they were able to translate the data into information and action for improvement. But has their underlying message of analyzing and translating data into information for the purpose of systems-level improvement been readily and widely accepted within health care? Why is it still a struggle today to examine and use data in our clinical practices for improvement? See Sidebar 5-1, right, regarding challenges to collecting data. How can providers partner with patients and families to assess and improve outcomes?

# Building Measurement Knowledge

Although the act of measuring health care processes and outcomes has increasingly become an integral part of the health care experience, most health care professionals (clinical and administrative) do not receive sufficient grounding in measurement methods and statistical applications to cope adequately with the growing demands to collect and analyze data for improvement. At some point, most health care professionals may have taken a class on introductory statistics, but overall there is relatively shallow knowledge in measurement principles and statistical methods used in health care improvement.

Many challenges exist along the measurement journey,[4] and it is not a particularly easy journey. With the growth of EHRs and pay for performance in many systems, data are now so common that many in health care are drowning in data. The challenge is that not all the measures are useful, and health care professionals do not learn how to use or act on data. Measurement can be time-consuming and feel like added work. It can be challenging to make sure data are accurate and consistent. Often we feel there are too many indicators or not the appropriate indicators for the work that we do. On top of this, measurement may feel

SIDEBAR 5-1

## What Is Measurement? What Are Measures in Health Care?

**Measurement** is the act or process of ascertaining the extent, dimensions, or quantity of something, while a **measure** refers to the unit or standard by which something is assessed.[1,2] Measurement often involves assigning a number (quantitative value) to some concept. Measures and measurement are ubiquitous in society, whether it is the star rating on apps and websites, public polls prior to elections, or the statistics about your favorite sports team and players. **Data** is the term used for the values of the measures (the "numbers" themselves, referred to as **quantitative data**), but data are not limited to numbers. Data also may be quotes or text that someone writes in an evaluation or gives during an interview. These are termed **qualitative data**.

In health care, measures, measurement, and data (both quantitative and qualitative) have exploded over the past decade. Electronic health records (EHRs) and Web-based interfaces make it easier to gather data, but simply gathering data does not make it understandable or actionable. Transforming data into actions requires an understanding of how and why the data were collected, a clear connection to the processes and context of the system (*see* Chapter 4), and skill in drawing valid conclusions from the data.

### References

1. Merriam-Webster. Measurement. Accessed Nov 22, 2017. https://www.merriam-webster.com/dictionary/measure.
2. Merriam-Webster. Measure. Accessed Nov 22, 2017. https://www.merriam-webster.com/dictionary/measurement.

threatening. If data are gathered and not used—particularly not used to inform decision making—then many become disillusioned with the measurement process. The best of intentions for collecting data and using measurement becomes muddled and ineffective in the frontline microsystems of care.

There are many tremendous potential benefits of measurement for improvement of care. When done right it can help you make decisions and make you feel more confident about the reliability of the care processes. Measurement allows you to keep tabs on what is going on and thus sets the stage for improvement of systems. In discussions with clinical and management colleagues, measurement can provide a common frame of reference and help them focus on what is important. Finally, measurement moves us away from anecdotes (individual case stories or $N = 1$) and one person's view to a more comprehensive view of the functioning of the system.

Measurement efforts can be traced back to the fundamental principles of the scientific method.[5] The scientific method is an iterative, circular process of starting with a hunch, a question, or a hypothesis. In clinical improvement work, this often manifests as the specific aim for the improvement work (see Chapter 3). Measurement allows the improvement team to assess the baseline functioning of the system and spot a possible quality gap and to determine whether instituted changes result in improvement. The results lead to a new hunch or modified hypothesis, new changes, and continued assessment of the processes and outcomes of the system. You can then see how measurement is integral to the scientific method, and while it is only one component, getting the measurement correct is a key element of strong, sustainable improvement.

# Fundamental Approaches to Measurement

All too often, health care professionals ignore the iterative, circular nature of the scientific method and view measurement as if it were a singular event—and as if the same methods can be applied in all approaches to measurement. Nothing could be farther from the truth. Solberg and colleagues provide a strong starting point for thinking about different approaches to measurement.[6] They point out that there are three fundamental facets to measurement in health care: research, accountability, and improvement.

"We are increasingly realizing not only how critical measurement is to the QI [quality improvement] we seek, yet how counterproductive it can sometimes be to mix measurement for accountability or research with measurement for improvement."[6(p. 137)]

The characteristics of each of these approaches to measurement are depicted in the rows of Table 5-1 on page 73. These aspects are basic requirements of any measurement approach. Each cell of this table describes how each aspect is applied for improvement, accountability, and research. Let's look at the columns individually to get a better understanding.

## Research as a measurement approach

The basic aim of research is to develop new generalizable knowledge or to test existing theories for the purpose of discovery. Researchers use elaborate methods to make sure the study design controls for exogenous variables that may create confounded results (outcomes due to extraneous variables rather than the interventions or study variables). Experimental designs provide the most control and therefore maximize the validity and reliability of the results. Researchers often collect more data than is needed in the event that reviewers, journal editors, or critics raise questions about the results or methods.[6] Statistical analysis for research uses biostatistics, a branch of statistics that compares groups or that identifies the factors influencing outcomes. The biostatistics in research measurement often produces a $p$ value and confidence intervals, which help us interpret the overall effect of the intervention as opposed to change from other factors. Measurement for research is an extremely important domain that essentially addresses the question of efficacy.[7] In everyday terms, research allows us to figure out what is effective and likely to work.

## Accountability as a measurement approach

Administrators, policy makers, clinicians, and others use measurement for accountability to compare outcomes of aggregate data between countries, states, or hospitals. It is typically summary data in a table that focuses on making comparisons between groups and asking a simple question such as, "Is performance better now than it was the last time?" or "Which region has the highest rate of childhood vaccinations?" In most instances, the answer is based on performance of the observed units against fixed targets or goals. Accountability data are usually descriptive and do not routinely include statistical analysis.

**TABLE 5-1** The Characteristics of the Three Types of Measurement in Health Care.

| Characteristic | Research | Accountability | Improvement |
|---|---|---|---|
| Aim | New generalizable knowledge | Comparison, choice, reassurance spur change | Improvement of processes and outcomes |
| Observability of Testing | Blinded or controlled | No test, observe current performance | Tests are observable |
| Bias | Design to eliminate bias | Measure and adjust to reduce bias | Accept consistent bias |
| Sample Size | "Just in case" data to have as much as possible | Obtain 100% of available data | "Just enough" data with small sequential samples |
| Flexibility of Hypothesis | Fixed hypothesis | No hypothesis | Hypotheses are flexible and change as learning takes place |
| Testing Strategy | One large test | No tests | Sequential tests |
| Determining If a Change Is an Improvement | Hypothesis testing, statistics (*t*-test, chi-square test, ANOVA, *p* value) | No change focus | Run charts or statistical process control charts |
| Confidentiality of Data | Research subjects' identities protected | Data available for public consumption and review | Data used by those involved with the improvement |

**Source:** Adapted from Solberg LI, Mosser G, McDonald S: The three faces of performance measurement: Improvement, accountability, and research. *Jt Comm J Qual Improv.* 1997 Mar;23(3):135–147.

## Improvement as a measurement approach

Finally, measurement for improvement focuses on monitoring the outcomes of a system over time to understand if the processes are efficient and effective.[8] We use measurement to determine whether or not interventions have had significant effects on the performance and outcomes of a system. It may also focus on how the processes relate to outcomes for patients. Measurement for improvement shares characteristics with measurement for research and accountability, yet it also has important unique components. Traditional research helps us determine "the what" while improvement allows us to determine "the how"

in a particular context (for example, How can we implement an efficacious idea, technique, procedure, or drug so that it performs reliably every time?). A major distinction between improvement measurement and the other two types of measurement in Table 5-1 is that improvement often incorporates statistical process control methods (which we'll discuss in detail in Chapter 6) to determine if there has been a significant change in performance. Statistical tests of significance (for example, *t*-tests, chi-square tests, logistic regression) are not typically appropriate for improvement, whereas analysis of the variation over time is the most important determinant of improvement.

## Navigating the Interfaces of Measurement Approaches

Health care organizations need leaders and frontline individuals who are comfortable and competent in being able to blend the three approaches to measurement. Although some might express that it can be counterproductive to mix the three approaches,[6] we do not view the three approaches as silos. These approaches are not independent and unrelated but rather are three facets of measurement. Health care leaders will improve their overall measurement capacity when they are able to navigate the interfaces of each measurement approach. Sometimes an individual can become strongly invested in only one approach to measurement. A person may talk about measurement for research as the "only" valid approach to measurement. Similarly, others may focus only on measurement for accountability such as aggregate data that compare hospitals, cities, or regions. Health care institutions need individuals who can function as translators of these three approaches to measurement—who speak the language of each domain. For health care professional leaders, this is a critical skill. To understand the valid, reliable, and solid measurement within each domain they must be able to move comfortably across the columns in Table 5-1 and not rely solely on one measurement silo.

### Translating across the measurement domains

An example will help to show you how serving as a translator and moving between the three facets of performance measurement can be very beneficial. The Dartmouth Atlas of Health Care uses data from the US Centers for Medicare & Medicaid Services, the US federal health insurance program for individuals over age 65, to document local, regional, and national variation in outcomes and resources (see http://www.dartmouthatlas.org).[9] The Dartmouth Atlas demonstrates geographic variation in aggregated outcomes, and many use it to compare performance from one locale or region to another. Table 5-2 on page 75 shows an example of comparison, aggregate data from the Dartmouth Atlas of 2014. You will notice some variation in the scores state to state in each of the three conditions. No one state is highest in any one condition. These aggregated data at the state level have an important utility for understanding accountability and differences between regions; however, aggregated data are of limited use for improvement within an individual state. For example, you might notice that Texas has a lower mammography rate. But these data are from 2014 and represent such a large geographical area it may be difficult to take action on this level of data. Aggregated data

presented in tabular formats or with summary statistics do not help you measure the impact of process improvements or redesign efforts, particularly those at the microsystem level. Aggregated data are useful for accountability, not for local improvement.[6]

## Understanding Variation in Measurement for Improvement

Because improvement of systems is the goal of our work in this book, we need to discover the unique benefits about measurement for improvement. W. Edwards Deming was a US physicist and statistician who worked in post–World War II Japan. He was a consultant to rebuilding industry in Japan after the war and has received much credit for the high quality of manufactured products. His work was translated to health care applications in the mid-1980s by Donald Berwick, MD; Paul Batalden, MD; and others, and it became the foundation for much of the modern QI movement in health care. One of Deming's classic statements related to measurement and improvement is: *"If I had to reduce my message for management to just a few words, I'd say it all had to do with reducing variation."*[10(p. 57)]

Understanding variation is vital to all improvement work. Let's take a practical example from the work of Carey and Lloyd[8] to show how recognizing the type of variation in the data can help you take action on a system.

### Variation in data and taking action.

Mary and Bill are both placing shots on a target (*see* Figure 5-3 on page 76). Who is the better shot? Mary's shots are clustered together, but none hit the bull's-eye. Bill's shots are more scattered, but he did hit the bull's-eye once. A more appropriate question would be, "What does each person need to do to hit the bull's-eye consistently?" It appears that Mary would merely need to adjust the sight of her rifle to the left and down slightly, while Bill may need to totally rethink his approach to shooting. His shots exhibit a random pattern on the target. Perhaps he was shooting outside and there was a swirling wind? How might he improve? If he adjusts his sight downward for his highest shot and gets it closer to the bull's-eye, he will force the lowest shot on the target farther away from the bull's-eye. This example demonstrates why understanding the underlying variation in a system is so vital. If you are sincere and passionate about understanding where your processes and outcomes have been, where they are now, and where they are headed in the future, then gaining knowledge about the type of variation and how to take action is key.

**TABLE 5-2** Sample Data from the Dartmouth Atlas of Health Care

| State | Mammography every 2 years, women age 67–69 | At least one primary care clinician visit in past year | Beta-blocker after heart attack |
|---|---|---|---|
| Alabama | 63 | 83 | 83 |
| California | 60 | 73 | 80 |
| Colorado | 60 | 77 | 84 |
| Missouri | 63 | 80 | 85 |
| New Hampshire | 71 | 78 | 89 |
| New York | 62 | 73 | 86 |
| Ohio | 61 | 79 | 85 |
| Texas | 58 | 78 | 82 |

This sample of *Dartmouth Atlas* data (http://www.dartmouthatlas.org) compares outcomes from eight states for three different conditions. The score in each cell represents the percentage of the Medicare population (age > 65) who successfully received the intervention in 2014; range is 0% (low) to 100% (high).

**Source:** Adapted from The Dartmouth Atlas of Health Care. Trustees of Dartmouth College.

## Potential consequences of not understanding variation

If you fail to account for variation and understand its role, you can be tempted to misinterpret the data and overreact to individual data points. Consequences of not understanding the variation in your data and its impact include the following[8]:

- You will be tempted to see trends where there are no trends.
- You will try to explain natural variation as special events.
- You will blame and give credit to others for things over which they have little or no control.
- You will have a distorted understanding of the process that produced the data.

Unfortunately, in health care we demonstrate these behaviors on a regular basis. For example, it is not uncommon when we receive and review our data to state, "These data are not reliable, valid, or accurate for my patients, my system, or my organization." We are very good at denying the data, distorting the process that produced the data, or blaming the individual or organization that delivered the data. We do this by claiming that our patients are sicker, older, or more complex, or that the time has lagged so much that the data are not relevant anymore. Sometimes this response is grounded in the belief that others should not be reviewing our performance in the first place. At other times, it is because we know that our results are either not particularly good or show a great deal of variation. Finally, it may be due to the fact that we have no idea what the variation is that lives in our data. Irrespective of the motivating factors, without a clear understanding of the variation in our processes and outcomes, it is very difficult to provide reliable results or make improvements.

## Example of Understanding Variation Within a Set of Data

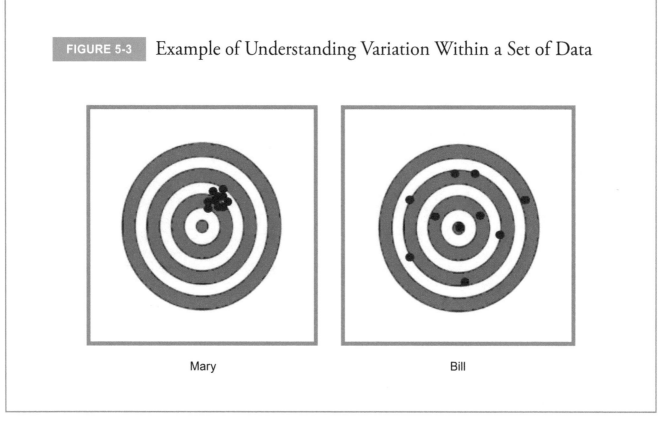

Mary                                         Bill

The data here are the individual shots on target by each person, Mary and Bill. Each makes 10 shots at the target.

Source: Carey RG, Lloyd RC. Measuring Quality Improvement in Health Care: A Guide to Statistical Process Control Applications. Milwaukee, WI: ASQ Press, 2001. Used with permission.

## What improvement measurement should be

In summary, measurement for improvement guides us in how to take action on the system. This is distinct from measurement used for research or accountability. Improvement measurement should be characterized by comprehensive, balanced data collection and analysis. We should be evaluating local systems and knowing whether the changes made led to improvements. Measurement for improvement seeks to understand the process and outcomes in relation to the specific causes (that is, the context of a health care setting). Simply stated, measurement for improvement provides a basis for decision making (*see* Sidebar 5-2, page 77). In Chapter 6, we will delve into the types of variation, how to use analytic tools to analyze variation, and how to link measurement to improvement strategies.

# Identifying a Balanced Set of Measures for Improvement

*Inez Anton is a family physician who recently received a summary of data about her clinic's patients with diabetes. The report card shows a mixed bag: the rate of yearly eye exams is higher, average hemoglobin A1c levels are higher than last year, and blood pressure control looks better than last year. The report card is an extraction of data from patient charts and the hospital lab system. It is summarized in a table with comparisons to "exemplary performers" in the region. Over lunch the next day, she expresses her frustration at these outcomes and shares the report with Tomas Vucic, the practice administrator, and Marla Edissen, the senior nurse in the clinic. Inez comments that this is ridiculous, as the data do not compare to clinics that are similar. She says, "This 'report card' is exasperating . . . who chooses these measures? I recognize our practice can get a bonus payment for good performance, but who makes these measurement decisions?"*

**SIDEBAR 5-2** Experiential Learning

When you use data for improvement and to make decisions, you engage in a common cycle of experiencing and learning. David Kolb's experiential learning cycle describes this process in more detail[1] (*see* Figure 5-4, page 78). We engage in this process when we care for an individual patient and when we work on system level improvement. We start at the top of this diagram with a concrete experience. Recall that in this chapter's opening vignette, one of the team's patients had an unanticipated wound infection. The surgical team, led by the pharmacist Tiffany's question, reflected on what this one case could mean in terms of the overall care of surgical patients. This is what we see on the right-hand part of Kolb's diagram. Tiffany made an abstract generalization (bottom of the diagram) when she asked whether wound infections were a common occurrence at the hospital. Teresa, the attending physician, initially dismissed this question, saying that wound infections are part of the usual course of practice.

This is where we get to the left-hand side of Kolb's model. Elizabeth Larsen, the nurse on the team, was ready to start testing the implications of a wound infection and the reliability of the timing and duration of preoperative antibiotics. She helped to further explore this hypothesis by obtaining outcome data about wound infections on the unit. This combination of the data and the hypothesis led to the initiation of an interprofessional team to identify the processes involved for perioperative antibiotic delivery. Our patient in the vignette, Annette Quinn, will likely recover from her infection and return home; however, the increased hospital stay, pain, and costs were unnecessary and could be avoided in the future if the team and the surgical microsystem can learn from its data to improve its outcomes and processes. Adding a patient to the improvement team ensures that the patient's point of view and in-depth experience in the system is part of the considerations for changes.

Kolb's model provides an opportunity to take our individual reflections—those things we notice during the delivery of care—and learn from them by identifying underlying concepts and generalizations. These are then used to test changes in the system. For our vignette, this might be an automatic EHR order for antibiotics or may evolve into a complete preoperative order set. This cycle of learning is core to improvement work and is similar to the scientific method. Analysis of data provides the vital role of assessing and testing our generalizations and understanding about the systems in which we work.

**Reference**
1. Kolb DA. *Experiential Learning: Experience as the Source of Learning and Development.* Englewood Cliffs, NJ: Prentice-Hall, 1984.

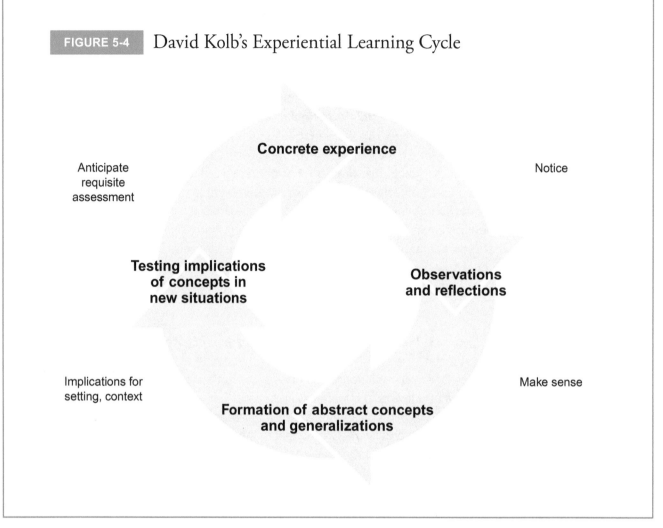

FIGURE 5-4    David Kolb's Experiential Learning Cycle

**Concrete experience**

Anticipate requisite assessment

Notice

**Testing implications of concepts in new situations**

**Observations and reflections**

Implications for setting, context

Make sense

**Formation of abstract concepts and generalizations**

"Testing implications of concepts in new situations" is the key step leading back to concrete experiences. Analytic data evaluation is an important part of this when applying Kolb's cycle to learning about systems. The level of data collection must align with the level of the system that is being considered.

**Source:** Kolb DA. *Experiential Learning: Experience as the Source of Learning and Development.* Englewood Cliffs, NJ: Prentice-Hall International, 1984. Printed with permission.

*Tomas and Marla look at the report and are just as perplexed. Marla states that their patients seem quite satisfied with their care: "We get very few, if any, patient complaints." Tomas comments that the EHR that started last year can provide trending data and analysis. He hasn't had the time to do this, and the information technology support group from the hospital has been too busy putting out fires in the new system to perform any data extraction. Once again, here is a system with lots of promise but little to show for it.*

*Together they realize that there must be a nugget of reality buried in these report cards, but they are unsure how to study their local processes to improve care for their patients with diabetes. Inez recalls that Dan Leibowicz was in the clinic for*

*a diabetes check-up a week ago. His diabetes control had been much improved over the past six months. "I wonder why he has made so much progress? I make the same recommendations to him as I do to others." Marla says, "We should ask him to work with us. I bet he can provide insights into what might be effective changes to make and what really adds value to diabetes care for patients." They agree this is a great idea . . . Marla will invite Dan to join the improvement team.*

Before you can display and interpret your data (and understand the variation in it), you must identify appropriate measures for the system. As we noticed in the vignette, sometimes measures are simply thrust upon us. A hospital or a health plan (insurance company) may recommend (or require) that a practice start measuring certain processes or outcomes. A health plan may even "score" a practice based on these measures. Examples of these measures might include readmittance rate to the hospital for patients with congestive heart failure, adequate blood pressure control for patients with diabetes, or rates of immunizations. These measures are recommended—in fact, demanded—by external forces. This is the reality of our health care systems, and it might be a reasonable point from which to initiate improvement; however, these measures of accountability are often not enough to support a meaningful improvement.

## Identifying Appropriate Measures of Value

The opportunity to identify your own measures may be daunting but provides the chance to define specific—and balanced—measures that are most helpful to your improvement team. Usually, a set of balanced measures may include data that are provided to you and data that you obtain on your own. When you identify your own measures, you can focus on those items that are most important to your practice site, to your microsystem, and, most importantly, to your patients.

### The value equation

In short, value is equal to quality divided by cost (value = quality/cost). This value equation comes into play whether you are buying a toaster, choosing a new laptop, or deciding which orthopedic group will do your mother's hip replacement surgery. It is also apparent that "quality" can have many different components or domains. The important parts of quality will be different whether you are purchasing a product or working to improve the delivery of a service such as health care. Dividing quality into more specific domains can facilitate the identification of very specific measures for the improvement work. Table 5-3, below, shows one example of how "quality" can be divided into three separate domains: clinical outcomes, functional status of the patients or the system, and satisfaction of stakeholders (patients, families, physicians, nurses,

---

**TABLE 5-3** Domains of Value to Assist Brainstorming About Possible Measures for Improvement Work with Some Generic Examples.

| | | |
|---|---|---|
| | **Clinical outcomes** | • Mortality and morbidity<br>• Signs, symptoms<br>• Complications<br>• Diagnostic test results |
| **Quality** | **Functional status of patients or the system** | • Physical function<br>• Mental health assessment<br>• Social/role function<br>• Measures of health status (pain, vitality, perceived well-being) |
| | **Satisfaction of stakeholders** | • Patient, family, and caregiver satisfaction with health care delivery process<br>• Patient's perceived health benefits |
| | **Costs** | • Direct medical costs (co-pay, hospital services, medications)<br>• Indirect social costs (time lost from work, caregiver costs) |

**Source:** Adapted from Nelson EC, Batalden PB, Lazar JS, editors. *Practice-Based Learning and Improvement: A Clinical Improvement Action Guide*, 2nd ed. Oak Brook, IL: Joint Commission Resources, 2007.

pharmacists, administrators). Cost remains its own domain and can represent the direct costs of a service (for example, How much does a primary care visit cost?) or the indirect costs (for example, How much time is lost from school after pediatric patients have their tonsils removed?).[11]

## Step 1: Brainstorming to identify measures

The domains within the value equation can be used for brainstorming to identify potential measures. The team "walks" through each of the components and determines what might be important measures for that domain. For example, the clinical row might include mortality rates or lab test results that are important for the specific improvement project. The functional row can include physical or mental functioning of patients as well as efficiency or flow through a clinical area. Satisfaction is often broad to include patient, family, and staff satisfaction. Some proposed measures might not fit exactly on one row or another, and this is okay. It is better to get the measurement ideas out on the table so we can identify a comprehensive set of measures. The team will edit the measures in the next step.

Table 5-4 on page 81 is an example of a list of measures generated by the diabetes improvement team from our case vignette. Notice the aim statement at the top of the table. As discussed in Chapter 3, the aim statement keeps the improvement effort focused. Also, note that the measures are from different perspectives and different stakeholders: patients, family, and staff. The clinical row includes several measures such as average hemoglobin A1c, blood pressure control, eye exams, foot exams, and lipid control. The functional row has measures related to patient hypoglycemic episodes and the number of patients enrolled in exercise programs. The satisfaction row contains elements of patient and family satisfaction with the office staff, the clinician, and the hospital. Also included is staff satisfaction with care for patients with diabetes. The costs row contains both direct and indirect costs of diabetes. Direct costs are those that involve financial outlays such as medication expenses, hospitalization payments, and clinic copayments. Indirect costs include days lost from work due to complications of diabetes.

The measures in Table 5-4 are a combination of *process measures* and *outcome measures*. Process measures evaluate actions that are directed or known to influence the end result. For example, the percentage of patients who receive a foot exam is a process measure. Receiving a foot exam is not an outcome of diabetes but is an important process put in place to screen patients with diabetes for potential lesions on their feet. An *outcome measure* assesses the end result of a process (or several processes). Outcome measures are often considered more important because they are a representation of the consequences of the processes. In this example, an outcome measure might be the number of patients who require a foot amputation because of diabetes-related complications. It is the main outcome of interest, but it is far downstream and an infrequent occurrence to be the only measure that is used. A combination of process and outcome measures is a key component of balanced measures for improvement.

## Step 2: Narrowing the list from the possible measures

The list of measures in Table 5-4 is extensive, and it would be impractical for the team to measure and evaluate *all* of these items. The brainstorming step helps you identify *possible* measures. The team now needs to choose the measures it will use. Team members narrowed their choices to those most important and most related to their aim. These are indicated in Table 5-4 by being **bolded** and underlined. Because the percentage of patients with a hemoglobin A1c level less than 7.0% and systolic blood pressure less than 130 mmHg both have a strong correlation with excellent clinical outcomes for patients, the team chooses to use these as their clinical measures. The functional measure will be the number of patient-days with hypoglycemic episodes. The number of days with low blood sugar will need to be extracted from charts, but the team felt this could be a reasonable proxy for a patient's function at home and participation in work and leisure activities. The team also chose to focus on patient *and* staff satisfaction to gauge both sides of the clinical encounter. The team really wanted to assess the number of days missed at work related to diabetes, but these data were too challenging to obtain. The team members settled on the total number of office visits and average prescription medication changes for patients related to diabetes.

As you see in Table 5-4, the team started with 16 total possible measures and then narrowed them to the 8 most important ones for patients with diabetes in the clinic. This collection of measures may not be perfect but is a good place to start. Team members may drop or add other measures as their work on diabetes care continues.

## Step 3: Moving to operational definitions

The next step is to write operational definitions for each of the measures (*see* Table 5-5 on page 82). An operational definition is a specific, detailed description of the measure so that everyone (on the improvement team and outside the

**TABLE 5-4**　Example of Using the Domains of Value

**Aim:** Over the next 9 months, we will increase the control of blood glucose and blood pressure by 50% for our patients with diabetes mellitus while keeping the costs for our patients unchanged.

**Examples of Possible Measures**

| | | |
|---|---|---|
| **Quality** | **Clinical outcomes** | 1. <u>**Total # of patients with DM**</u><br>2. Average HbA1c for all patients<br>3. <u>**% patients with HbA1c < 7%**</u><br>4. <u>**% patients with systolic blood pressure less than 130**</u><br>5. % patients with foot exam<br>6. % patients with diabetic eye exam<br>7. # emergency department visits for diabetes-related concerns<br>8. % patients with low density lipoprotein less than 100 |
| | **Functional status of patients or the system** | 1. # patients enrolled in exercise program<br>2. <u>**Total # hypoglycemic episodes per month**</u> |
| | **Satisfaction of stakeholders** | 1. <u>**Patient satisfaction with provider, office staff, and hospital**</u><br>2. <u>**Staff satisfaction with care for patients with diabetes**</u> |
| **Costs** | | 1. <u>**Prescription medication costs**</u><br>2. <u>**# office visits per month**</u><br>3. Hospital charges<br>4. Days missed at work related to diabetes complications |

Example of using the domains of value for the team working to improve care for patients with diabetes. Bold/underlined items are the measures that the improvement team decided to use for the project. See text for full description. DM, diabetes mellitus.

**Source:** Adapted from Nelson EC, et al., editors. *Practice-Based Learning and Improvement: A Clinical Improvement Action Guide*, 2nd ed. Oak Brook, IL: Joint Commission Resources, 2007.

team) knows exactly *what* each measure describes. The operational definition often also includes where the data are generated and gathered (such as lab test and chart review), *who* is responsible for obtaining the data (for example, office staff, insurance plan, or outside firm), and *what* is to be included in a numerator or denominator. Although writing these definitions may seem laborious, the clarity they provide will be well worth the effort as the project progresses.

## Step 4: Qualitative or quantitative?

When it comes time to actually collect data for your measures, it is important to be clear whether you are building qualitative or quantitative measures. For example, staff satisfaction could be assessed with a lunchtime feedback session, similar to a "focus group" approach. In this case, a qualitative evaluation through structured discussion will provide greater depth of responses than a quantitative survey. This could be a convenient and nonthreatening opportunity for some directed feedback about the diabetes care. At other times, quantitative data

TABLE 5-5 Operational Definitions for the Measures
Identified in Table 5-4

| Measure | Operational Definition |
| --- | --- |
| Total # patients with DM | Total number of patients in our practice who carry diagnosis of diabetes mellitus (DM), type 1 or type 2 |
| % patients with HbA1c < 7% | Of those patients with DM who have had an HbA1c drawn in the past 12 months, the percentage (or proportion) who have a value less than 7 |
| % patients with systolic blood pressure < 130 | Of those patients with DM, the percentage (or proportion) of patients whose most recently recorded systolic blood pressure is less than or equal to 130 |
| Total % hypoglycemic episodes per month | Total number of low blood sugar reactions reported by all of our patients |
| Patient satisfaction with provider, office staff, and hospital | To be determined once we find a suitable satisfaction survey for our patients, and we will work with our patient partner to identify the core issues |
| Staff satisfaction with care for patients with diabetes | Major themes of DM care from the perspective of all members of our staff |
| Prescription medication costs | Total costs (not just co-pay) incurred each month for DM-related medications and supplies |
| Total # office visits per month | Total number of office visits per month that are coded for 250.XX (diabetes-related care) |

are more appropriate. For example, data that are gathered and reported quarterly by an insurance company or a governmental agency are typically quantitative in nature and consist of counts, percentages, rates, or scores. The time interval or frequency of each assessment is also important to consider. Values such as percentages of patients with systolic blood pressure less than 130 and percentages of patients with HbA1c less than 7.0% could be extracted monthly from the EHR (with assistance from the information technology staff). This would allow a quicker turnaround time for identifying whether or not a change in the care process makes a difference in the outcomes.

## Using Other Data Instruments or Collection Methods

Other data may require new instruments or collection methods. Although the practice in our vignette reports no patient complaints, how much do team members know about the overall satisfaction from their patients with diabetes? Including Dan or other patients on the improvement team will help the practice understand the patient experience and allow the patients to coproduce the diabetes care with the practice. With Dan's help and guidance, the team could use a standardized survey sent to diabetic patients to assess satisfaction. Perhaps the office staff would focus on more than the office microsystem or the patient-preceptor dyad and find ways to help patients in their personal care system (*see* the discussion in Chapter 4 regarding context and systems). Notice in Table 5-5 that the team does not have a way to assess patient satisfaction, so they are planning to enlist an outside agency to help survey their patients.

Importantly, no one piece of data provides the entire story of the clinical system under investigation, and not one of these measures is more important than another. Because the systems in which we work (and where patients receive care) are complex, a balanced set of measures can account for clinical outcomes, patient functional and satisfaction status, and costs. These measures—identified by using the value equation—help you assess the system and make decisions for improving many aspects of care.

# Displaying Measures for Analysis

After measures are chosen, it may be cumbersome to follow multiple measures in several electronic files or on many sheets of paper. Although it may not be possible for every improvement project, bringing the measures together into a comprehensive display as a data instrument panel, or dashboard, can be very helpful.[12]

## Data Dashboard

A data dashboard is better analogy for data display than a report card. While a report card conjures up visions of judgment on a specific task (pass/fail), a dashboard is intended to monitor and provide feedback on the state of the system, whether it's a car traveling along the highway or an office providing care to patients with diabetes. Figure 5-5 (page 84) is an example of a dashboard for diabetes care that is organized along our domains of value. Notice that the clinical data about the number of patients with diabetes and the two outcome measures are displayed in graphs. These are statistical process control charts, or more simply "control charts." These charts are one way to assess the variation in data, and we will cover them in more depth in the next chapter. For now, just recognize that each data point is a summary of monthly data, and each month when the data is extracted another point is added to each chart.

The functional data also have a control chart; however, because the team needed to gather the information about the number of low blood sugars per month, there are only a few data points on this chart. Each month, another data point will be added to the chart, so the information will grow as the amount of data grows. The satisfaction data contain a summary of the staff feedback about diabetes care and a note that patient satisfaction surveys have been received from three companies. The interprofessional QI team will need to decide which survey to use. Finally, the cost data are also noted in control charts. We can summarize from the EHR the prescription cost, broken down by types of medicines, and the number of office visits per month for diabetes.

This dashboard allows for a quick, overall assessment of the various measures. For example, perhaps the team recommends prescribing a new, expensive diabetes medication in hopes of increasing the percentage of patients whose A1c is < 7.0%. If the prescription costs start to rise with no concomitant increase in the percentage of patients under control, the team will be able to recognize this as it charts the data. This type of display demonstrates one of the tremendous benefits of multidimensional, balanced measures.

# Summary

Measurement alone is not sufficient for improvement, but it is one of the key steps in the Model for Improvement. Aggregate data in tabular format are best used for accountability but often lead to judgment, not improvement. Although summary data for accountability have a role in the comparison of systems, regions, or countries, they are limited in their utility for improvement. Measurement must focus on gaining insight into the processes and outcomes of the system.

Data analysis for improvement starts with identifying measures. The value equation is one structure that can help a team identify balanced measures for a project. By focusing on the value of care delivered, the team can address both the quality and the costs within the system. Although often there are more data and more measures than a team can reasonably handle, the team chooses which measures to use that will give the best overall assessment of the system it is trying to improve.

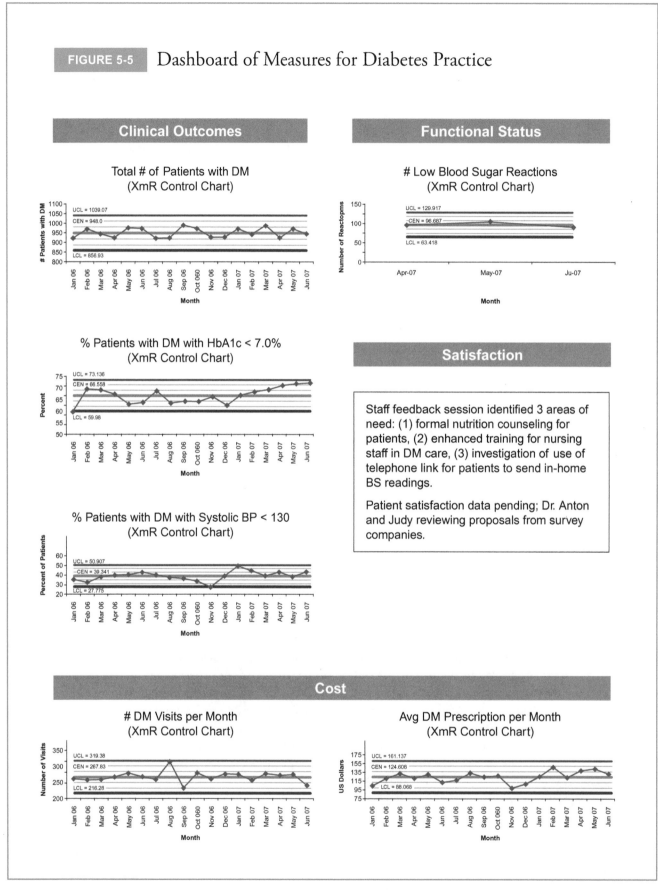

**FIGURE 5-5** Dashboard of Measures for Diabetes Practice

XmR Control Chart is a statistical method to assess the variation in a data set over a period of time. Control charts are explained in detail in Chapter 6. UCL, upper control limit; CEN, center line; LCL, lower control limit; DM, diabetes mellitus; BP, blood pressure; BS, blood sugar.

# Study Questions

A medical student and a nurse practitioner student are paired to work in a hemodialysis unit. Hemodialysis is the process of extracting fluid and solutes from the serum of patients with severe acute and chronic renal failure. Patients with chronic renal failure who require hemodialysis come to the unit three times per week to be dialyzed for three to four hours each time. At the end of the first week, the dialysis nurse manager invites the students to join in their hemodialysis quality improvement (HDQI) meeting.

In preparation for the meeting, the manager suggests that both students begin to pay attention to the processes and flow in the unit. The students notice that patients and staff arrive and are generally in good spirits each morning. By midday and into the afternoon, the mood on the unit changes considerably. Patients and family members are frustrated that the hemodialysis times are running late. Staff are working hard to make the flow better. Patients and family members state that they need to get back to work, and the time overruns are very inconvenient. The students talk with several patients who were scheduled for a three-hour dialysis run but are now close to four hours. One patient says he had just been in the hospital for a bloodstream infection that he suspects he got from the hemodialysis center. Another patient relates that she has a

temporary dialysis catheter because her arteriovenous graft was not mature enough when dialysis needed to start. The students can see that there are many opportunities for improvement in this unit.

At the HDQI meeting, the topic for the day is measurement. Much of the discussion focuses on the number of dialysis slots, how many patients are being served, and the recent financial statement. The nurse manager expresses his frustration at these one-dimensional data. He asks for some ideas about what else might be measured and what might be helpful for the unit's improvement.

1. Use the scenario above (and other information you may have about hemodialysis) and create a set of possible measures for the hemodialysis unit (*see* Table 5-6, below). Use the value framework described in the chapter to think broadly: It is a brainstorming opportunity, so be creative for each row in Table 5-6. Be sure to consider many perspectives (patients, families, clinicians) when creating measures. Write the possible measures in the cells of the right-hand column.

2. Take the measures from your table and write an operational definition for one measure from each row in Table 5-7, page 86. The operational definition is a specific and detailed description of the measure so that

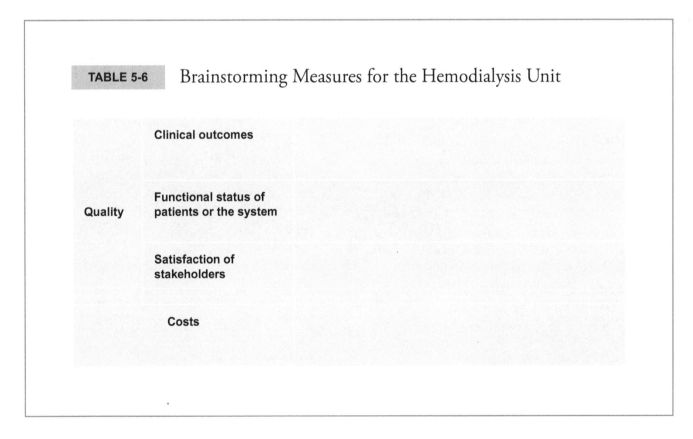

**TABLE 5-6**   Brainstorming Measures for the Hemodialysis Unit

| Quality | Clinical outcomes | |
| | Functional status of patients or the system | |
| | Satisfaction of stakeholders | |
| | Costs | |

| TABLE 5-7 | Operational Definitions for Hemodialysis Unit Measures |
|---|---|
| **Measure** | **Operational Definition** |
| Clinical outcomes | |
| Functional status of patients or the system | |
| Satisfaction of stakeholders | |
| Costs | |

everyone recognizes exactly what each measure describes. It might include where the data are generated and gathered (such as a lab test or a chart review) and who is responsible for obtaining the data (for example, office staff, insurance plan, or outside firm).

3. How might you consider displaying these data? With whom would you share them? Who will be on the improvement team?

## References

1. Agency for Healthcare Research and Quality, National Guideline Clearinghouse. Clinical Practice Guidelines for Antimicrobial Prophylaxis in Surgery. (Updated: Feb 1, 2013.) Accessed Nov 22, 2017. https://www.guideline.gov/summaries/summary/39533/clinical-practice-guidelines-for-antimicrobial-prophylaxis-in-surgery?q=antibiotics+before+colon+surgery.

2. Cohen I.B. Florence Nightingale. *Sci Am*. 1984 Mar;250(3):128–137.

3. Donabedian A. The end results of health care: Ernest Codman's contribution to quality assessment and beyond. *Milbank Q*. 1989;67(2):233–256.

4. Lloyd RC. Navigating in the turbulent sea of data. *Clin Perinatol*. 2010 Mar;37(1):101–122.

5. Lastrucci CL. *Scientific Approach: Basic Principles of the Scientific Method*. Cambridge, MA: Schenkman, 1967.

6. Solberg LI, Mosser G, McDonald S. The three faces of performance measurement: Improvement, accountability and research. *Jt Comm J Qual Improv*. 1997 Mar;23(3):135–147.

7. Glasziou P, Ogrinc G, Goodman S. Can evidence-based medicine and clinical quality improvement learn from each other? *BMJ Qual Saf*. 2011 Apr;20 Suppl 1:i13–17.

8. Carey RG, Lloyd RC. Measuring Quality Improvement in Health Care: A Guide to Statistical Process Control Applications. Milwaukee, WI: ASQ Press, 2001.

9. Trustees of Dartmouth College. The Dartmouth Atlas of Health Care. Accessed Nov 22, 2017. http://www.dartmouthatlas.org/.

10. Neave HR. *The Deming Dimension*. Knoxville, TN: SPC Press, 1990.

11. Nelson EC, Batalden PB, Lazar JS, editors. *Practice-Based Learning and Improvement: A Clinical Improvement Action Guide*, 2nd ed. Oak Brook, IL: Joint Commission Resources, 2007.

12. Nelson EC, et al. Report cards or instrument panels: Who needs what? *Jt Comm J Qual Improv*. 1995 Apr;21(4):155–166.

# Measurement Part 2: Using Run Charts and Statistical Process Control Charts to Gain Insight into Systems

 Objectives

**After reading this chapter, you will be able to do the following:**

1. Recognize the value of analyzing data over time by using run charts and statistical process control charts.

2. Describe the difference between common- and special-cause variation.

3. Interpret run and statistical process control charts.

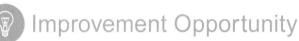 Improvement Opportunity

## Data Assessment

Jonah Mills has been a family physician in rural Idaho for more than 12 years. He recently assumed responsibility as medical director for three family medicine clinics. It has been a challenging transition. The clinics are located in different towns in the region, about 20–30 minutes from one another, and he has been trying to unify their approach to patient care. Today Jonah is meeting with the multisite quality improvement (QI) team, which includes nurses, physician assistants, a pharmacist, several patients, an office administrator, students, and other physicians, to review some data about the treatment for patients with chronic heart failure at all three facilities.

The three clinics initiated an electronic health record (EHR) system about one year ago. There was—as would be expected—a significant learning period to integrate the new technology into patient care. Initially, it was a challenge just to find information and enter it into patient charts. One advantage of this particular EHR system is that the software provider was able to download patient data from the prior system's lab and pharmacy records. Although the EHR system has been in use for only about a year, the database contains patient data from the past several years.

The team reviewed the data on patients with chronic heart failure. Although almost every patient has had an echocardiogram to assess left ventricular function, the pharmacist noted that there was a low rate of beta-blockers for patients with heart failure (*see* Table 6-1, page 88). Research evidence shows that the use of beta-blockers is associated with a significant increase in left ventricular function and a decrease in mortality. Jonah is not sure what to make of the data and asks the team, "When you look at these numbers from our three sites, which site has the 'best' outcomes? Who has made the most gains over the past year? Who needs the most help?"

| TABLE 6-1 | | | | Percentage of Patients with Heart Failure Who Received a Beta-Blocker |
|---|---|---|---|---|

| Month | Site 1 % | Site 2 % | Site 3 % | Month | Site 1 % | Site 2 % | Site 3 % |
|---|---|---|---|---|---|---|---|
| Jan-15 | 61 | 64 | 53 | Jan-16 | 66 | 64 | 64 |
| Feb-15 | 68 | 65 | 50 | Feb-16 | 65 | 63 | 68 |
| Mar-15 | 65 | 61 | 51 | Mar-16 | 66 | 61 | 69 |
| Apr-15 | 70 | 65 | 49 | Apr-16 | 67 | 61 | 70 |
| May-15 | 62 | 56 | 51 | May-16 | 68 | 60 | 69 |
| Jun-15 | 65 | 59 | 52 | Jun-16 | 72 | 59 | 68 |
| Jul-15 | 60 | 66 | 53 | Jul-16 | 80 | 58 | 67 |
| Aug-15 | 66 | 68 | 55 | Aug-16 | 67 | 61 | 69 |
| Sep-15 | 68 | 60 | 58 | Sep-16 | 65 | 59 | 68 |
| Oct-15 | 65 | 66 | 64 | Oct-16 | 61 | 58 | 68 |
| Nov-15 | 61 | 69 | 66 | Nov-16 | 64 | 59 | 70 |
| Dec-15 | 65 | 66 | 65 | Dec-16 | 63 | 57 | 67 |
| 2015 average % | 65 | 64 | 56 | 2016 average % | 67 | 60 | 68 |

# QI Measurement: Evaluating Systems over Time

Chapter 5 discussed the historical developments of measuring outcomes in clinical care and also provided tools for identifying measures for a clinical system. This chapter focuses on using methods to analyze data in health care to gain insight into the functioning of the system—data for improvement (*see* Table 5-1, page 73). In this chapter, we will focus on robust and dynamic methods of measurement intended to monitor systems for changes that occur and to predict what will happen in the future: the run chart and the statistical process control (SPC) chart, also known as a control chart.

Measurement for improvement is unique from other forms of measurement. Unlike most comparative statistics, we use measurement for improvement not to identify differences between groups (static, one point in time) but instead to monitor systems over time (dynamic, continuous measurement). Most comparative data analyses look backward and reflect on what has been measured in the past, like looking in the side mirror in a car (*see* Figure 6-1, right).[1] While these analyses provide a sufficient summary of where you have been, they provide only a slight view of what lies ahead (perhaps like looking around the edges of the side mirror). In contrast, analyzing data over time—with the use of run charts and control charts—offers a much different perspective; it is like looking through the front window of a car while driving (*see* Figure 6-2, right). When you are looking through the front window, the mirror provides a panoramic view of the road behind; however, you also see a clear view in front of you, in anticipation of the road ahead. Similarly, analyzing data over time can identify how a system is currently operating as well as predict future functioning of the system. These tools provide a statistically powerful method to understand what is happening in a system.

For example, imagine that an improvement team in the intensive care unit is evaluating the outcome of the initiation of a bundled intervention to reduce ventilator-associated pneumonia (VAP).[2] A bundle is a group of evidence-based interventions that are known to improve outcomes and should be implemented together for maximum effectiveness. The team began implementing the VAP bundle in January 2015. In January 2016 the chief quality officer wants to know whether the bundle intervention has made a difference. The team uses two approaches: comparative statistics using

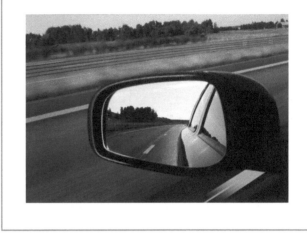

**FIGURE 6-1**

## Comparative Statistics

Comparative statistics provide a clear view of past performance. As with a side rearview mirror in a car, you mostly see the road behind, with a bit of the road ahead around the edges.
Source: Photo by Gregory Ogrinc.

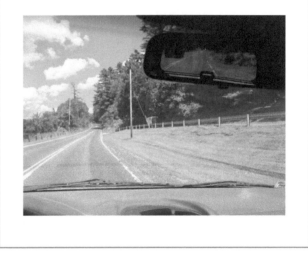

**FIGURE 6-2**

## Analysis of Data over Time

Examining data over time (run charts and control charts) provides a view of past performance with an expectation about future performance. Like a view out the front window of a car, you see the road ahead as well as a clear picture of what is behind.
Source: Photo by Gregory Ogrinc.

before-and-after data of average number of infections and monthly data displayed on a run chart. The comparative summary statistics in Figure 6-3 on page 90 demonstrate a decrease from an average of seven infections per month in

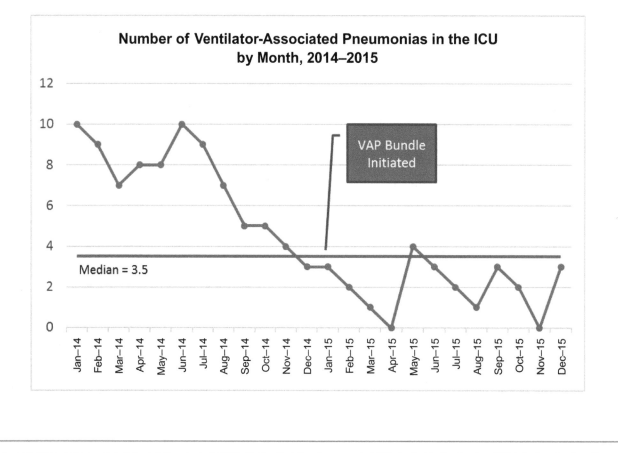

**FIGURE 6-3** Comparison of Yearly Summary Data (Table) and Monthly Data Graphed over Time for Ventilator-Associated Pneumonia (VAP) in the Intensive Care Unit

Evaluation of Ventilator-Associated Pneumonia in the ICU, 2014–2015.

| Year | Total Number of VAP | Monthly Average VAP |
|------|---------------------|---------------------|
| 2014 | 85 | 7 |
| 2015 | 24 | 2 |

**Number of Ventilator-Associated Pneumonias in the ICU by Month, 2014–2015**

Median = 3.5

VAP Bundle Initiated

The bundle intervention was initiated at the start of 2015. Notice that the decrease in VAP started in September 2014, before the bundle was initiated. ICU, intensive care unit.

2014 to an average of two infections per month in 2015. Such a dramatic change (even without running a specific statistical test) is encouraging. However, when the team uses a dynamic display of monthly VAP data in a run chart, it is clear that that the reduction in VAP started prior to the bundle implementation (note the trend that started in July and August 2014). It appears that since the intervention of the bundle, the rate of VAP has been steady. The improvement team notes that further analysis may be needed to determine whether the bundle was effective in maintaining the lower rate of infections. Perhaps the bundle helped the unit reach zero infections in April and

November 2015? As we discovered in Chapter 5, summary data in a static, tabular format is not effective for assessing the impact of interventions.

# Run Chart and Statistical Process Control (SPC) Charts: The Basics

A defining characteristic of QI is to show that the strategy for change (which is often multifaceted) works to bring about a measurable and sustained difference in process or outcome. Two-point, before-after studies are a weak demonstration of change, such as in the table in Figure 6-3. Strong demonstration of change in a system overcomes the limitation of before-after analysis by capitalizing on the concept of *replication*. Replication, or the process of evaluating successive, sequential data points, creates confidence that the intervention produces the pattern of change observed in the results. Run charts and control charts (SPC) use the principle of replication for analysis to demonstrate whether a change has occurred from preintervention (baseline phase) to postintervention (implementation phase) and through multiple successive interventions. These are within the family of time-series analyses that plot multiple points, with each point representing the operationally defined unit of measurement (such as a daily, weekly, or monthly proportion; or mean; or time between events).[3]

## Analyzing Why a Significant System Change Occurs

When a run chart or an SPC chart contains at least 14 data points, the statistical probability of detecting a significant change in the data (a "signal" from an increase or decrease in performance, an unusually high or low point) is less than 5% (equivalent to a *p* value < 0.05). This is based on probability statistics of replication, which generate power from point-to-point variation to detect a signal. So, when a signal appears in a chart, it is the same power as a *p* value < 0.05 that occurs in comparative statistics. These methods can detect that a statistically significant change has occurred in a system, but the team must identify *why* it has occurred: a new process, reaction to a change to the system, stress to the system from an external source (for example, many staff out sick). Evaluating a system with these tools identifies *what* has occurred in the system and gives the team the opportunity to gain insight into *why* the system responded as it did.

## How Run Charts Work

A run chart displays data in a time-ordered sequence (*see* Figure 6-4 on page 92) and can easily be constructed with graph paper and a pencil. We plot time along the *x*-axis and the appropriate scale for the data along the *y*-axis. Time on the *x*-axis may be days, months, or quarters, or may consist of consecutive measurements (for example, blood sugar, blood pressure) taken over some time period, even if not done at regularly spaced intervals. The body of the run chart contains each value in consecutive order connected by a line. As the data are plotted on the run chart, a measure of central tendency is also added. For a run chart, the measure of central tendency is the *median*, the point at which half of the data points are above the line and half of the data points are below the line. For example, in a run chart with 25 data points (*see* Figure 6-4), we would draw the median line at a location where 12 data points are above the line and 12 data points are below it (the median is 121 in this example). We can use run charts for any process and with any type of data, such as whole numbers, percentages, and proportions.

## How Statistical Process Control (SPC) Charts Work

An SPC chart uses the point-to-point variation in the data to derive control limits. The most essential type of SPC chart is called an XmR chart, which uses the average as the measure of central tendency (*see* Figure 6-5 on page 93). Upper and lower control limits (UCL and LCL) represent boundaries that are about three standard deviations on each side of the average. We can calculate these using a formula that includes the average of the data points (x), the average of the difference between each data point (R), and a constant (2.66). This formula is represented as follows:

$$UCL = x + 2.66*R$$
$$LCL = x - 2.66*R$$

Thus, as each new point is added to the chart, the average, UCL, and LCL are updated. This is the important dynamic characteristic mentioned earlier in the chapter. Because these calculations change with each point that is added, we usually construct control charts with the help of software.

The basic anatomy of an SPC chart is similar to a run chart. We represent time on the *x*-axis, and data values on the *y*-axis. Individual data points are plotted in the body of the figure. The average and the control limits are derived from the data. The data in Figure 6-5 are the same as in the run chart in Figure 6-4, but notice that the average in the SPC chart is nearly 125, while the median in the run chart is 121. The added power of an SPC chart comes from the

FIGURE 6-4a Anatomy of a Run Chart

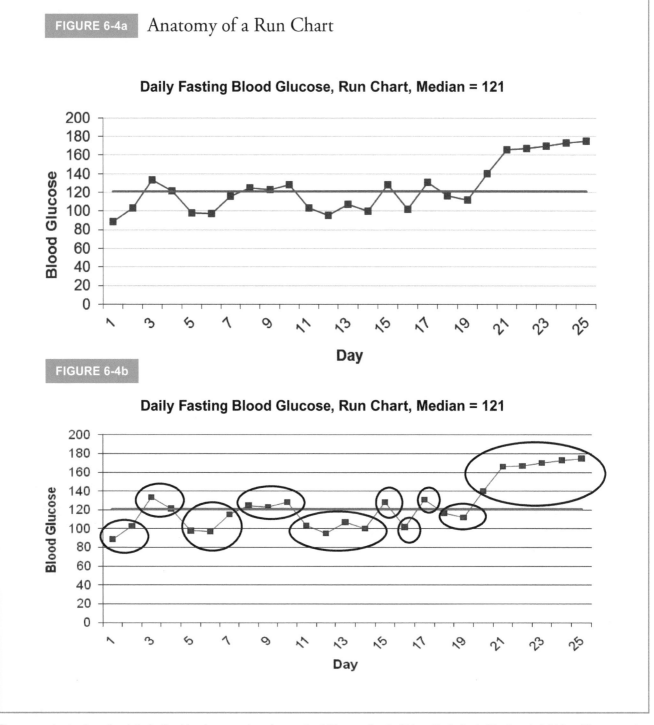

**Daily Fasting Blood Glucose, Run Chart, Median = 121**

FIGURE 6-4b

**Daily Fasting Blood Glucose, Run Chart, Median = 121**

These run charts show the daily fasting blood sugar values for a patient. The median is 121 and is indicated by the straight line. The second chart shows the 10 runs circled.

upper and lower control limits, which are approximately 162 and 88 in Figure 6-5. These control limits provide the parameters that we use to gain insight into the variation in the data.

# Common- and Special-Cause Variation

Whether using run or SPC charts to represent data, determining the type of variation present in data is a vital step in gaining insight into the system characteristics and taking the correct action to improve the system. There are two types of variation to understand: common-cause and special-cause variation. *Common-cause variation* is considered inherent in the process and due to regular, natural, or ordinary causes. It is always present in a system, and we can consider it to be the baseline variation in a system. Common-cause variation originates from all of the steps of a process and, when present on its own, results in a stable process we can consider as predictable. Common-cause is also called random or unassignable variation. *Special-cause variation* is due to effects that are usually outside the steps of the process. It affects some, but not necessarily all, aspects of the process and results in an

unstable, unpredictable process. Special-cause variation may also be referred to as nonrandom or assignable variation.

Common-cause variation does not mean "good" variation. It means only that the process is stable and predictable. Similarly, special-cause variation does not mean "bad" variation. A special cause may represent a very good result, which you might want to enhance. *Special cause* merely means that something has affected the process to make it unstable and unpredictable.

For example, imagine that you are seeing a patient with high blood pressure who is measuring his pressure at home every day. Over the course of two weeks, his systolic blood pressure ranges from 158 to 173 mmHg. These 14 days of data would indicate entirely common-cause variation. The blood pressure is stable and predictable, and the data contain only common-cause variation; however, it is entirely unacceptable because his goal for his systolic blood pressure is less than 140 mmHg. Now let's introduce an antihypertensive medication into his routine. Over the course of several days, the systolic blood pressure drops to between 125 and 140 mmHg. This would be considered a special-cause variation since it is a significant disruption to the system—but it is a good special-cause variation. The

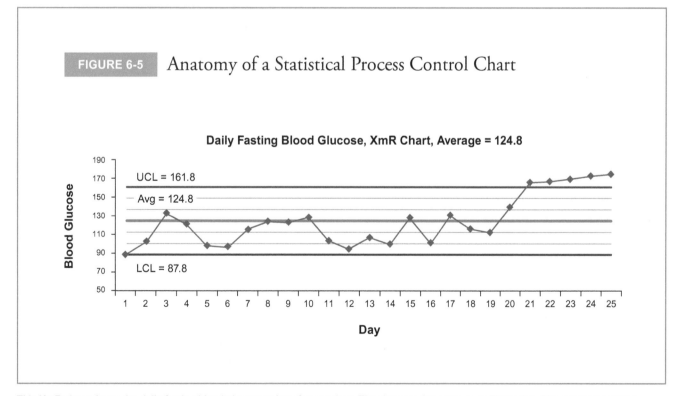

**FIGURE 6-5** Anatomy of a Statistical Process Control Chart

This XmR chart shows the daily fasting blood glucose values for a patient. The data are the same as in Figure 6-4. The average is 124.8 (green line), and the upper control limit (UCL) is 161.8, while the lower control limit (LCL) is 87.8.

blood pressure self-care system for this patient at this point in time is considered unstable and unpredictable even though it has been moved closer to the clinical goal. After taking the new medication for one month, it is likely that he will have only common-cause variation in his systolic blood pressure readings again, but now with his blood pressure at the clinical goal of less than 140.

## Implications of Differences in Causes of Variation

The key point is that knowledge of the aim of the improvement (Chapter 3), the process, the context, and the system (Chapter 4) helps you identify whether or not the outcomes are acceptable. In measurement for improvement—whether for high blood pressure in an individual patient or in the percentage of patients in a microsystem with controlled high blood pressure—the measures become part of the feedback process and can also influence the changes in the system.

Determining special- or common-cause variation has profound implications as to whether and how you should take action on a system. Recall in Chapter 5 how understanding the variation in Mary's and Bill's target shooting guided how each would change her or his sighting scope to hit the bulls-eye consistently (*see* Figure 5-3, page 79). Understanding the type of variation in your data (and thus in your system) directs you to take appropriate action on the system (*see* boxes with check marks in Table 6-2, below). If action is needed in a system, and you indeed take

action, this is the appropriate step to take. Similarly, if action is *not* needed, and action is *not* taken, this is also appropriate. Systemic losses in efficacy and efficiency occur when action is needed but not taken. This leads to loss of efficacy and efficiency from passivity. Similarly, if action is *not* needed, but is taken—for example, many changes are made to a process without understanding the underlying variation—the system may experience a loss of efficacy and efficiency from tampering. Understanding the variation in the data over time leads to better improvement and substantial insights into the process, which leads to more effective change.

# Interpreting Run and Statistical Process Control Charts

Using a run chart is the simplest way to analyze data over time. In many ways, the run chart is the forerunner of the SPC chart. Either type of chart can assist in determining the type of variation present in a system, but in some ways, a run chart is similar to a plain x-ray, while an SPC chart is similar to a CT (computed tomography) scan. The x-ray is often easier to obtain and interpret but gives less information than a CT scan. Sometimes an x-ray is all that is needed to make a diagnosis; however, at other times, the additional time, detail, and expense of the CT scan is required for the appropriate diagnosis and treatment of a patient. Similarly, a run chart may be appropriate for a simple and

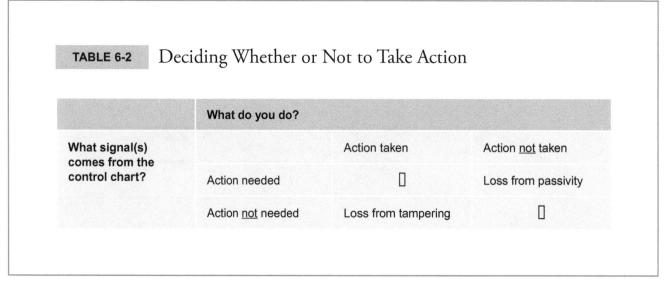

| TABLE 6-2 | Deciding Whether or Not to Take Action | | |
|---|---|---|---|
| **What signal(s) comes from the control chart?** | **What do you do?** | Action taken | Action <u>not</u> taken |
| | Action needed | ☐ | Loss from passivity |
| | Action <u>not</u> needed | Loss from tampering | ☐ |

Examining data over time with a run chart or statistical process control chart will help determine whether action is needed. Taking action on a system that is stable is tampering and will likely lead to loss of efficiency and effectiveness. Similarly, *not* taking action on a system that is out of control is passive and leads to a loss of efficiency and effectiveness.

FUNDAMENTALS OF HEALTH CARE IMPROVEMENT ❖ THIRD EDITION

straightforward analysis of a system, but sometimes an SPC chart is needed for more detailed and in-depth analysis.

Interpreting each run and SPC chart aids us in understanding the variation that lives in the data. There are rules of detection to identify whether special-cause variation is present in each chart. If none of the rules are fulfilled, then the chart indicates only common-cause variation. These rules are based on probability that certain patterns would not occur by chance alone. Let us look at each of the basic rules of detection and illustrate with a few examples.

## Rules of Detection in Run Charts

A run chart should have at least 14 points for sufficient power to draw conclusions. The example in Figure 6-4 (page 92) has 25 points of daily fasting blood sugar data for a patient with diabetes, so there is adequate power to proceed with interpretation. After the chart is created, we apply three rules of detection to each run chart to determine whether or not the chart shows any of the following special-cause signals:

1. Too few or too many runs, which is an assessment of the overall variability in the data
2. A shift in the process with seven or more consecutive points on one side of the median
3. A trend of seven or more points continually increasing or decreasing

The presence of any one of these indicates a change in the data (and a change in the process that the data represent) that is statistically significant.

Special-Cause Signal #1—Indication of overall variability: We determine too few or too many runs by counting the number of runs on the chart. A *run* is a group of successive points (or even one point) on one side of the median. If a point falls on the median, it is not counted as part of a run because it does not add further information about variability in the data. The number of runs is an estimate of the overall variability in the data, determined from probability statistics, and is found in a statistical table that provides the low and high expected number of runs based on the total number of points in a chart (*see* Table 6-3, right).[4] A chart with 25 points should have between 9 and 17 runs. If there are fewer than 9, it would be a special-cause signal of too little variability. If there are more than 17, it would be a special-cause signal of too much variability. The second example in Figure 6-4 has each run circled. There are 10 runs total, so the amount of overall variability is appropriate—no special cause from test #1.

**TABLE 6-3**

## Determining the Expected Number of Runs

| Number of data points not on the median | Lowest run count | Highest run count |
|:---:|:---:|:---:|
| 12 | 3 | 10 |
| 13 | 4 | 10 |
| 14 | 4 | 11 |
| 15 | 4 | 12 |
| 16 | 5 | 12 |
| 17 | 5 | 13 |
| 18 | 6 | 13 |
| 19 | 6 | 14 |
| 20 | 6 | 15 |
| 21 | 7 | 15 |
| 22 | 7 | 16 |
| 23 | 8 | 16 |
| 24 | 8 | 17 |
| 25 | 9 | 17 |
| 26 | 9 | 18 |
| 27 | 9 | 19 |
| 28 | 10 | 19 |
| 29 | 10 | 20 |
| 30 | 11 | 20 |

Special-Cause Signal #2—Indication of a shift in the process: The second test is for a shift in the process. A shift occurs when there are 7 or more consecutive points on one side of the median. There are no shifts in Figure 6-4.

Special-Cause Signal #3—Indication of a trend:
The third test is for a trend, which is indicated by at least 7 consecutive points increasing or decreasing. One increasing trend is present in Figure 6-4, from day 19 through day 25 indicating a signal of special-cause variation.

## Determining the reason the variation has occurred

Although a run chart can identify the variation, it does not tell you why this has occurred. For example, we identified a trend in Figure 6-4a, indicating a special-cause signal that something has perturbed this patient's self-care system for diabetes. To determine why this has occurred, we need to turn to the process of care for this patient. Upon further investigation, we find that this patient was on vacation and was not able to follow his diabetic diet while traveling. He ate more sweets and carbohydrates during that time period. The run chart gives us the power to identify that the change in dietary intake was significant enough to cause a real, statistical change in the patient's fasting blood sugar. This was not just a slight "bump" from being on vacation but rather indicates a significant change to his self-care system.

## Rules of Detection in Statistical Process Control Charts

An SPC chart also should have at least 14 points for sufficient power to draw conclusions; however, the upper and lower control limits provide additional ways to test for special causes of variation. In statistical process control charts, we don't count runs because the width of the control limits (distance between the upper and lower control limits) estimates the overall variability. Very wide control limits indicate more variability than narrow control limits. We identify special-cause variation in a control chart when one of the following occurs:
1. A single point falls outside a control limit.
2. A shift occurs in the process with seven or more consecutive points on one side of the median.
3. A trend of seven or more points continually increases or decreases.

After we plot the data on a control chart (using the formulae from page 91 or computer software), we apply the rules for detecting special-cause variation. The control chart in Figure 6-5 (page 93) is an XmR type chart (sometimes called an "Individual's" or "I-chart") that contains the same trend from day 19 through 25 that we observed in Figure 6-4. There are no shifts in the control chart; however, with the addition of the control limits, we can identify a special-cause signal on the third point of the trend on day 21.

This is the first point outside the control limits. Had we observed these points as they occurred each morning, we could have identified a significant change in the patient's fasting blood sugar (on day 21) several days earlier with the control chart than with the run chart (on day 25, the seventh point in the trend).

## Acting on Interpretations from the Charts

The run and SPC charts are tools to help us focus on taking the correct action. The action for this individual patient is guided by the insight garnered from the charts. The patient and his health care team now aware that vacations are a time when he needs more support for his diabetes care. Perhaps a refresher session with a diabetic dietary counselor about healthy eating while traveling would be helpful. Maybe he requires a short-term increase in his medications. The special-cause signal directs specific actions to bring the system into control to meet the goal.

But what if there were no special-cause signals? The interpretation would then be that the chart shows only common-cause variation. The action to address common-cause variation is quite different. Instead of addressing specific issues such as dietary intake while on vacation, the provider and patient would examine the overall system performance, determine whether the patient is meeting his goal for diabetes care, and, if he is not at goal, then address the underlying processes of his diabetes care. If he were at goal, then no changes would be the appropriate course of action.

## Using Statistical Process Control Charts to Predict Future Performance

Another advantage of the control chart is that the control limits can help predict future performance (see Figure 6-5). Over the past 25 days, the upper and lower control limits for this patient's fasting blood sugar are between 87 and 162. Using the predictive characteristics of a control chart, we anticipate this person will have a fasting blood sugar between 87 and 162. When we add each value to the chart, the control limits adjust; this is the dynamic property of a control chart. The chart's continual updates account for the new information that arrives with each new data point. Although this patient can anticipate fairly good blood sugar control (between 87 and 162 fasting blood sugar), as soon as the 164 blood sugar occurs on Day 21, the chart would prompt the patient to realize that this is unusual, so he can then determine the cause and take action.

Demonstrating Common- and Special-Cause
Variation

One way to examine the difference between common-cause variation and special-cause
variation is with a classroom exercise designed by Dr. Paul Miles. He handed out 22
1.69-ounce packages of candy-coated chocolates to a group of students (one bag to each
student), claiming that the students could use statistical process control to predict the
number of green candies in each bag. He asked each student, one by one, to open the
package and count the number of green candies. Using a spreadsheet, he created a run
chart of the data (see Figure 6-6a, page 98). When all 22 students had submitted their data,
Miles calculated the control limits for the data and produced an XmR control chart (see
Figure 6-6b, page 98). The control limits are parameters within which the students could then
predict the number of green candies in the unopened packages. The students then opened
5 more bags of candies and, sure enough, the number of green candies in Packages 23
through 26 fell within the predicted range of 4 to 18 (the lower and upper control limits of
3.9 and 17.8, respectively). The interpretation of these charts (see Figures 6-6a and 6-6b)
indicate only common-cause variation. There are no special-cause signals. The system for
green candies in a package is stable and predictable.

Next, Miles presented a 1.69-ounce package of holiday candies containing only green and
red candies. That package contained 25 green candies. The addition of the holiday package
to the series is an example of a special-cause variation. It indicates a change in the
underlying production process (that is, the underlying system). Figure 6-6c (page 99) shows
the addition of bags 23–26 and the holiday bag (point #27). This point is above the upper
control limit, indicating that there is special-cause variation. In this case, the reason for the
special-cause signal is obvious, a different production of candies for the holidays. As you will
see later, identifying special-cause variation directs you to examine the process and system
from which the data arise to identify the source of the special cause.

## Control Limits for Groups of Data

Another feature of the SPC chart is that we can use control
limits for groups of data in a chart. In other words, one
chart may have data with two or more sets of control limits.
For example, to evaluate the effectiveness of an intervention,
control limits for the process before the intervention can be
set to remain constant, and new control limits can be
recalculated reflecting the time after the intervention is
implemented. This is called *splitting the control limits*.
Another example of this process is when a run of data is
outside of the control limits. The data prior to this special-
cause variation can be set to remain constant and new

control limits calculated (*see* continuation of the vignette
starting on page 99 for an example of where this would be
appropriate). Splitting and recalculating control limits helps
us determine when special-cause variation becomes stable at
a new level (that is, it now becomes new common-cause
variation), another example of the dynamic nature of SPC.

## XmR Control Charts

There are many different types of SPC charts. The most
common is the XmR chart (Individual's chart, or I-chart).
It is robust enough to be used with any type of data. In
addition to XmR charts, other specific control charts are

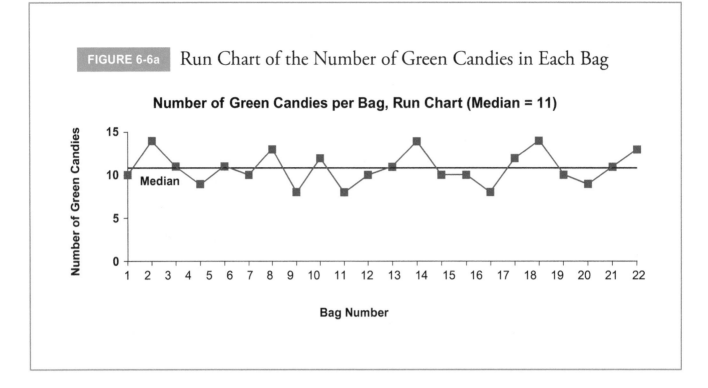

**FIGURE 6-6a**  Run Chart of the Number of Green Candies in Each Bag

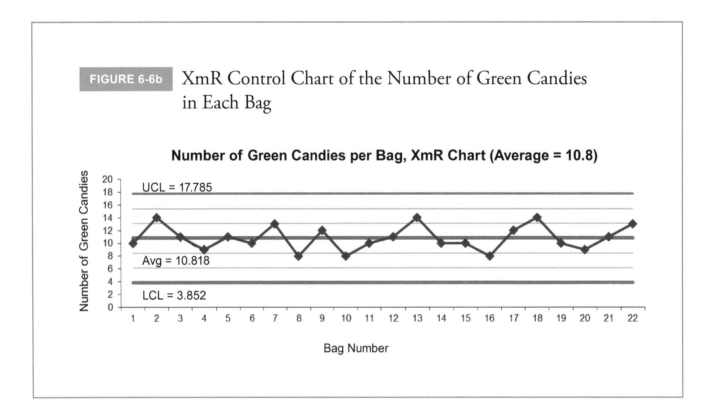

**FIGURE 6-6b**  XmR Control Chart of the Number of Green Candies in Each Bag

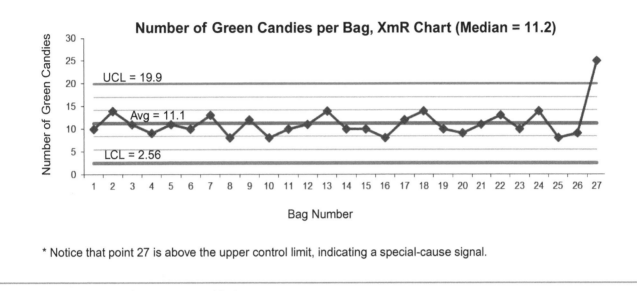

**FIGURE 6-6c** XmR Control Chart of the Number of Green Candies from a Holiday Package of Candies*

**Number of Green Candies per Bag, XmR Chart (Median = 11.2)**

*Y-axis: Number of Green Candies*

UCL = 19.9
Avg = 11.1
LCL = 2.56

*X-axis: Bag Number*

* Notice that point 27 is above the upper control limit, indicating a special-cause signal.

UCL, upper control limit; LCL, lower control limit.

used depending on the underlying distribution of the data (normal, binomial, geometric). The calculations used in the XmR chart make it rigorous enough to be used with any data that have any underlying distribution. While other types of charts might be more technically appropriate for percentage or proportion data, an XmR chart is valid for plotting any data. For more detailed information about control charts in health care settings, see the article by Amin[5] or the books by Carey[4] and Provost and Murray[6] listed at the end of this chapter.

*Now let's return to our example of the improvement team concerned about the low rate of administration of beta-blockers for patients with heart failure to see how these concepts come together. The team comments that it is difficult to determine which site is performing best using the available data. In Table 6-1 on page 88, it appears that beta-blocker usage at Site 2 was about the same as that at Site 1, but it declined a bit in 2016. Site 3's performance was well below the other two sites in 2015, but it seemed to make a rather spectacular improvement of 12 percentage points the following year. The team suggests using run and control charts to use all the data for the past 24 months.*

*Jonah Mills has the data in two formats. First the team examines the data using run charts (see Figures 6-7a–6-7c). Although Table 6-1 shows that Site 3 had the best performance in 2016, the team agrees that, according to the run charts, much of that site's improvement occurred more than 14 months ago! They apply the rules for detecting special-cause variation and find too few runs in the chart for Site 3 (only two), which indicates a special cause occurring at Site 3. Similarly, Site 2, which initially had a similar performance to Site 1 but then declined, shows a trend that occurred from November to July. This is also a special-cause signal, and the process that produced that result should be investigated. Finally, Site 1 remained just about the same over the 24 months. There was a peak in July 2016, but on the run chart there is only common-cause variation. The team summarizes its analysis in a table (see Table 6-4, page 101).*

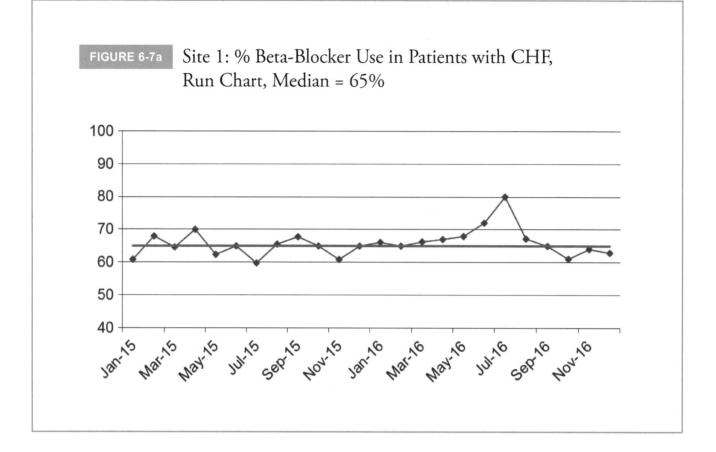

FIGURE 6-7a  Site 1: % Beta-Blocker Use in Patients with CHF, Run Chart, Median = 65%

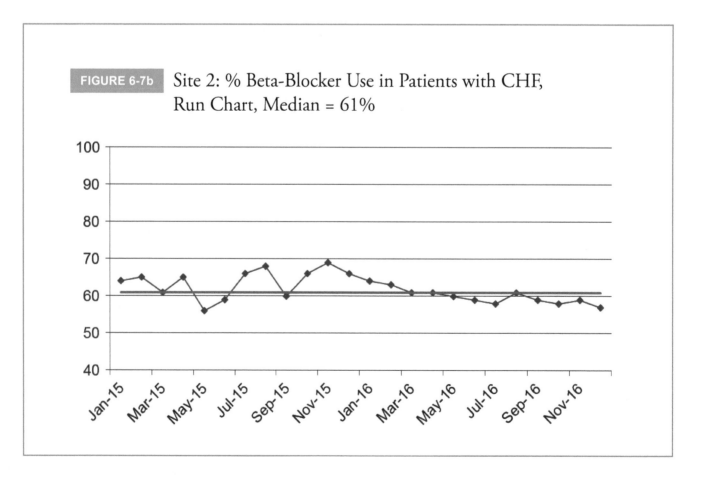

FIGURE 6-7b  Site 2: % Beta-Blocker Use in Patients with CHF, Run Chart, Median = 61%

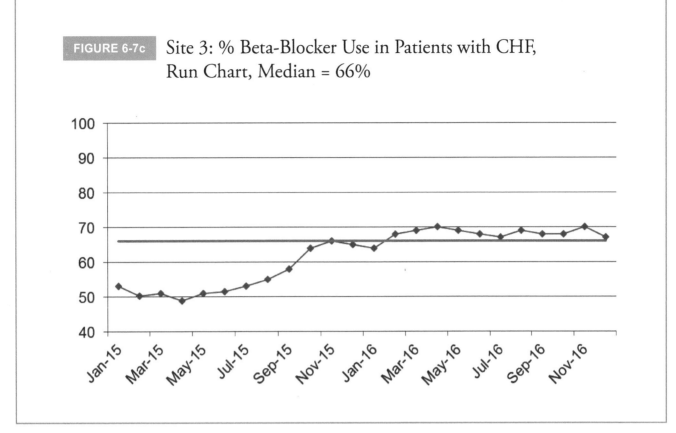

**FIGURE 6-7c**  Site 3: % Beta-Blocker Use in Patients with CHF, Run Chart, Median = 66%

Run charts of the percentage of beta-blocker use by patients with congestive heart failure (CHF) by site from 2015 through 2016.

**TABLE 6-4**  Summary Interpretation of Run Charts from Sites 1–3

| Site | # Runs | Shift? | Trend? | Interpretation | Action |
|------|--------|--------|--------|----------------|--------|
| 1 | 9 | No | No | Common-cause variation | Will need to examine fundamental process of beta-blocker prescribing. |
| 2 | 6 | No | Yes | Two special-cause signals | Investigate the trend to determine why the decrease in performance occurred at that time. |
| 3 | 2 | Yes | Yes | Three special-cause signals | Investigate all three signals to determine why the site has leveled off in performance. |

This table summarizes the improvement team's analysis of the data from Sites 1–3 (Figures 6-7a–6-7c). From Table 6-3 (page 95), the expected number of runs is between 8 and 17.

Jonah is impressed with the team's analytical ability, and he turns now to the XmR control charts, which contain the same data (see Figures 6-8a–6-8c, this page and next page). Examining the data using the control charts, the team notices that Site 1 had a special-cause signal in July 2016. Site 2 has the same trend seen in the run chart and also shows a shift (March 2016–September 2016). Site 3 is the most striking, and nursing student Kaitlyn Smith states, "This is interesting [pointing at Figure 6-8c]: Site 3 did so much better after they implemented an intervention in October 2016 to improve beta-blocker use. But it seems that the effect was limited, and the system has been stable since then. It's hard to see with the control limits as they are drawn. Can we adjust the chart to make this change more apparent?"

Jonah appreciates Kaitlyn's insight and shows the team a chart with the control limits split and recalculated (see Figure 6-8d, page 104). "Essentially, the system has remained stable for the past 14 months. It now has an average of 67% of patients receiving beta-blockers, but the width of the control limits tells us that Site 3 can expect to operate anywhere from 63% to 71% in the future unless something is done to change the system. Kaitlyn comments, "It's unfortunate that Site 3 made such good progress but then leveled off and has not continued to improve the system since October 2015."

Jonah pauses and considers the other XmR charts (see Figures 6-8a and 6-8b). "In many ways," he says, "this is equal cause for concern. Site 2 had some episodes of increasing its numbers, but the past 12 months have seen a decrease, with 10 consecutive months under the center line. It is concerning that the system has taken a downward turn, and this should be addressed soon. Site 1 is also interesting: in July 2016, it reached 80% of patients. This is above the upper control of 76%, so it is a special-cause signal. I wonder what happened that month to get such good results? And why the decline since then?"

He continues, "We've all been trying hard to improve and have shown some successes. These charts help us to identify where the changes have made a real difference and how we might amplify their successes and perhaps reverse trends where the outcomes are not as strong as we want." The team agrees and determines that the next step is to meet with the individual clinic directors and the chronic heart failure patients at those clinics to better understand what is happening at each site. The team then summarizes its findings from the analysis in a table (see Table 6-5, page 105).

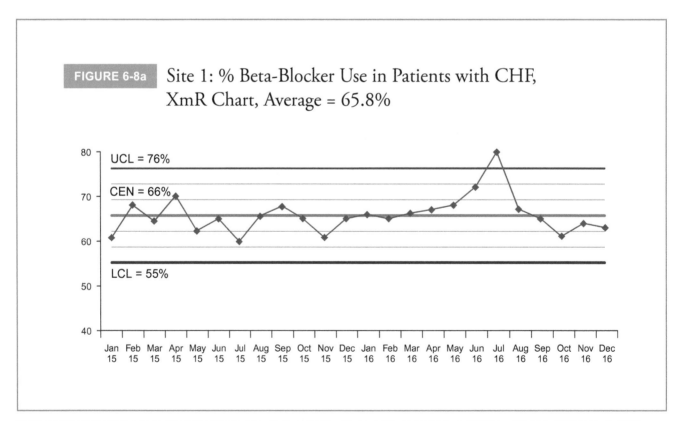

**FIGURE 6-8a** Site 1: % Beta-Blocker Use in Patients with CHF, XmR Chart, Average = 65.8%

XmR control charts of the percentage of beta-blocker use by patients with congestive heart failure (CHF) by site from 2015 through 2016. UCL, upper control limit; CEN, center line; LCL, lower control limit.

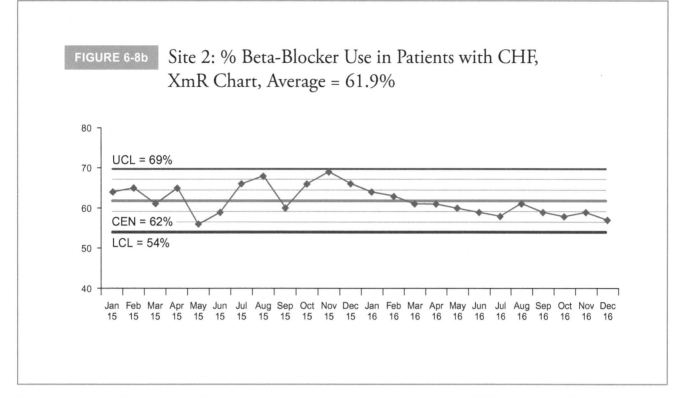

XmR control charts of the percentage of beta-blocker use by patients with congestive heart failure (CHF) by site from 2015 through 2016. UCL, upper control limit; CEN, center line; LCL, lower control limit.

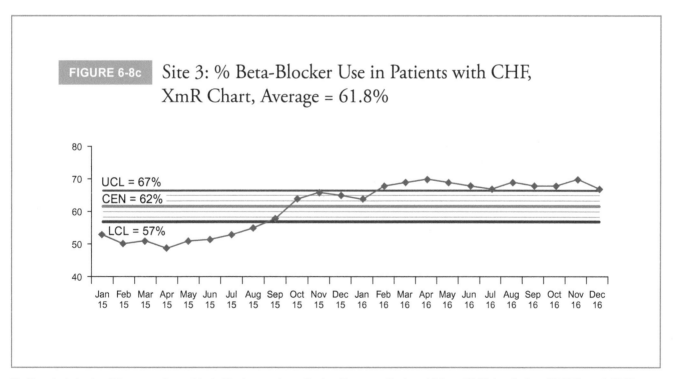

XmR control charts of the percentage of beta-blocker use by patients with congestive heart failure (CHF) by site from 2015 through 2016. UCL, upper control limit; CEN, center line; LCL, lower control limit.

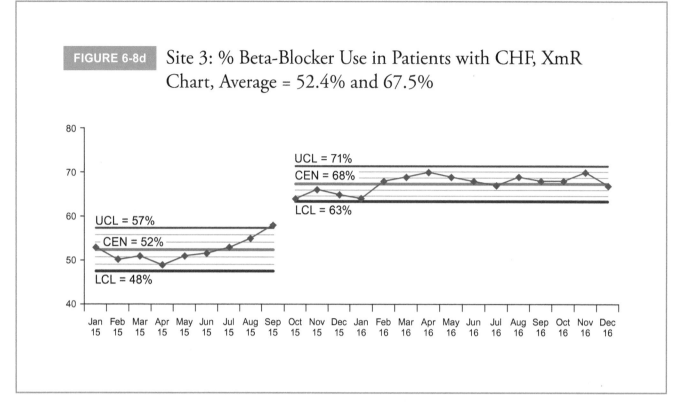

Site 3: % Beta-Blocker Use in Patients with CHF, XmR Chart, Average = 52.4% and 67.5%

XmR control charts of the percentage of beta-blocker use by patients with congestive heart failure (CHF) by site from 2015 through 2016. UCL, upper control limit; CEN, center line; LCL, lower control limit.

## Summary

A defining characteristic of QI is to demonstrate that the strategy for change works to bring about a measurable difference in process or outcome. Measurement for improvement monitors systems and processes over time (dynamic, continuous measurement); whereas comparative statistics are usually used by researchers to identify differences between groups (static, cross-sectional). The two main measurement tools are run charts and statistical process control (SPC) charts. Run and control charts use the principle of replication to demonstrate whether a change has occurred from preintervention (baseline phase) to postintervention (implementation phase).

Applying the rules for interpretation determines whether the variation in the process is common cause or special cause. These rules include identification of runs, trends, and out-of-control points. The interpretation of this variability directs action on the processes of a system. Measurement for improvement and the interpretation of the variability in processes or outcomes are keys to the success of QI efforts in health care.

## Study Questions

You are a member of your unit's cardiothoracic surgery QI team. Surgery has always been fascinating to you, and heart and lung surgery is the most interesting of all. You enjoy the clinical work, and this hospital is a new member of a regional consortium that is focused on improving all aspects of their coronary artery bypass grafting (CABG) surgeries. What an opportunity to combine your love of surgery as a discipline and learn to improve care for surgical patients!

Throughout the first week, you notice that the team waits for a serum potassium level before the patient can come off the heart-lung bypass machine. This is important because patients who are on the bypass machine for a longer period have more complications. In the first six cases this week, it has taken between 12 and 40 minutes for the "stat" potassium level to be reported by the lab. Everyone in the operating room (OR) "knows that the lab is slow," but you wonder what is really happening with this process?

One morning later that week, the first case of the day for your team is canceled. Instead of catching up on some reading, you decide to follow a "stat" potassium sample from the other OR to the lab and back. You make some

| | | | | | | | |
|---|---|---|---|---|---|---|---|
| **TABLE 6-5** | | | | Summary Interpretation of the XmR Control Charts from Sites 1–3 (Figures 6-8a to 6-8d) | | | |

| Site | LCL | UCL | Points outside the control limits? | Shift? | Trend? | Interpretation | Action |
|---|---|---|---|---|---|---|---|
| 1 | 55 | 76 | One | No | No | One special-cause signal | Investigate the point above the UCL from July 2010. What went right this month? |
| 2 | 54 | 69 | No | Yes | Yes | Two special-cause signals | Investigate the decreasing trend to determine why the performance changed and remained at a lower level. |
| 3 | 57 | 67 | Many | Yes | Yes | Three special-cause signals | Investigate all three signals as to why the site has leveled off in performance. |
| **Recalculated Control Limits** | | | | | | | |
| 3 | 48 | 57 | One | No | No | One special-cause signal | None, because it was in the distant past. |
| | 63 | 71 | No | No | No | No special-cause signals<br><br>Common-cause variation in past 14 months | Examine the fundamental process of beta-blocker prescribing. How can we move to even better performance? Why are we "stuck" at 67.5%? |

LCL, lower control limit; UCL, upper control limit.

notes and create the following deployment flowchart of the sample's journey (*see* Figure 6-9, next page):

You are amazed to see how much goes into the process. The sample is drawn from the patient in the OR and taken to the OR charge desk where the surgical clerk, who seems to do everything for everyone at the same time (and does a good job of it), calls for a transport. When it's in the chemistry lab, the sample is logged, run, and completed within about seven minutes. The lab has very clear records of this. The result is then telephoned back to the surgical clerk, who may or may not be able to answer the phone and relay the lab result to the OR right away. You draw curlicue-style lines to show where there are significant delays and

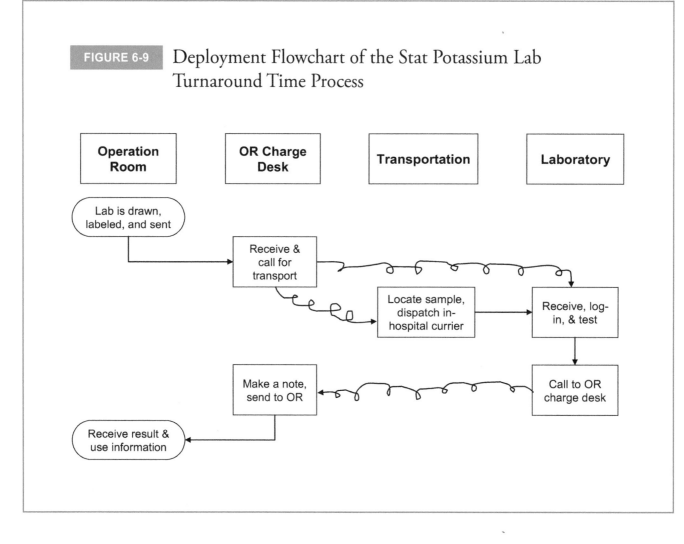

**FIGURE 6-9**  Deployment Flowchart of the Stat Potassium Lab Turnaround Time Process

variability in the process. Wow! What a complicated process for such a seemingly simple lab test!

You decide to get some data to evaluate this process, so you go back through the last 30 CABG cases and create a control chart of the number of minutes for the stat potassium to be reported to the OR. Your initial chart looks like the XmR chart in Figure 6-10 on the next page:

1. What does the information in this XmR chart tell you about the system?
   a. Are there any signals that indicate special-cause variation?
   b. What does it mean to have common-cause variation in this process?
   c. If no changes are made to the system, what is the range (low to high) that you anticipate it would take for the next stat potassium sample to be reported? How do you know this range?

After you review the process diagram and the chart with the team, everyone is impressed with your knowledge and assessment of the system. One of the nurse anesthetists recommends that the lab call directly to the OR instead of relaying the message through the surgical clerk. The lab agrees to try this change for a week, and stat potassium turnaround times from the eight cases that week are added to the XmR chart (*see* Figure 6-11, next page).

2. What has happened to the performance of the system?
   a. Are there any signals that indicate special-cause variation?
   b. Is the system functioning at its goal of a stat potassium turnaround time of less than 15 minutes? How do you know?
   c. What happened to the upper and lower control limits with these new data? Why?
   d. What else does this chart tell you?

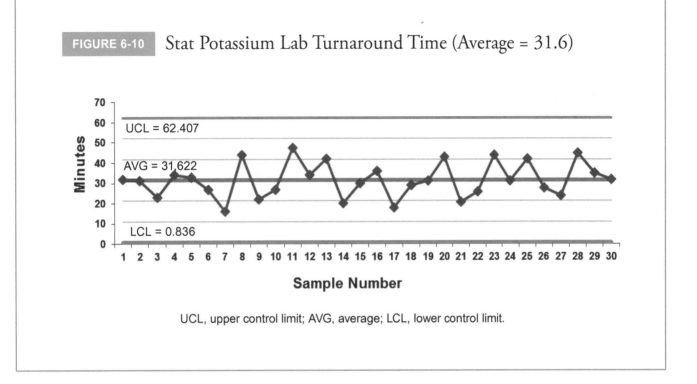

**FIGURE 6-10**  Stat Potassium Lab Turnaround Time (Average = 31.6)

UCL, upper control limit; AVG, average; LCL, lower control limit.

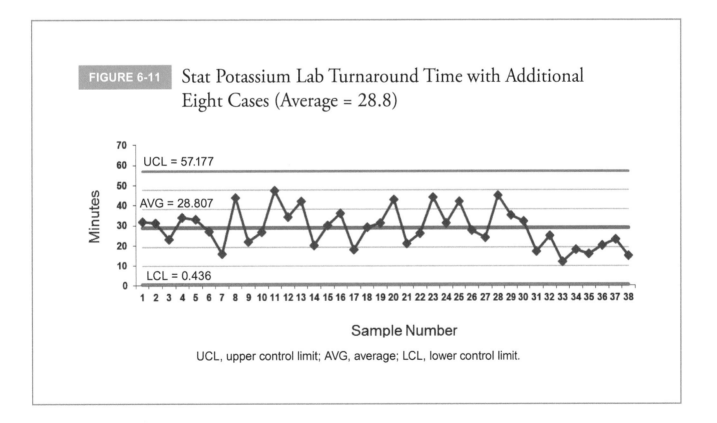

**FIGURE 6-11**  Stat Potassium Lab Turnaround Time with Additional Eight Cases (Average = 28.8)

UCL, upper control limit; AVG, average; LCL, lower control limit.

# References

1. Wheeler DJ. *Understanding Variation: The Key to Managing Chaos.* Knoxville, TN: SPC Press, 1993.

2. Rello J, et al. A European care bundle for prevention of ventilator-associated pneumonia. *Intensive Care Med.* 2010 May;36(5):773–780.

3. Ogrinc G, et al. The SQUIRE (Standards for QUality Improvement Reporting Excellence) guidelines for quality improvement reporting: Explanation and elaboration. *Qual Saf Health Care.* 2008 Oct;17 Suppl 1:i13–32.

4. Carey RG. *Improving Health Care with Control Charts: Basic and Advanced SPC Methods and Case Studies.* Milwaukee: ASQ Quality Press, 2003.

5. Amin SG. Control charts 101: A guide to health care application. *Qual Manag Health Care.* 2001;9(3)1–27.

6. Provost LP, Murray SK. *The Health Care Data Guide: Learning from Data for Improvement.* San Francisco: Jossey-Bass, 2011.

# Understanding and Making Changes in a System

 **Objectives**

**After reading this chapter, you will be able to do the following:**

1. Recognize that systems change occurs in a nonlinear, complex fashion.

2. Identify strategies for changing a clinical process to improve quality.

3. Appropriately use Everett Rogers's description of adoption of innovation to carry out a change in a system.

4. Describe the role and utility of the Model for Improvement and the Plan–Do–Study–Act (PDSA) cycle for testing small changes and for building knowledge about a system.

5. Identify barriers to change and strategies to overcome those barriers.

## Improvement Opportunity

### Patient Education

Bri'elle Wilson, a fourth-year medical student, is finishing her internal medicine outpatient rotation with physician Robert Jerome. She is ready to complete the rotation and move on to her residency interviews. She is looking forward to interviews for a general surgery residency and has been frustrated at what she perceives as the slow pace of outpatient general internal medicine.

She grabs the chart from the door of her next patient and scans the information. George Bernard is here for a hypertension follow-up. It has been challenging to get his blood pressure into the normal range over the past six months. He was initially 182/98. Robert, the physician, has added various antihypertensive medications from different classes, advised the patient on lifestyle changes, and increased several of the medications to maximum doses. Despite all this, Bri'elle notes that Mr. Bernard's blood pressure today is 156/86, still above the goal of > 140/> 90. She shakes her head in frustration, takes a deep breath to compose herself, knocks on the door, and enters the room.

Mr. Bernard is a 57-year-old welder who has been seeing Robert Jerome for about two years. Bri'elle introduces herself as a medical student, sits down, and says, "Thank you so much for coming today. I know you have been here about every six weeks or so, and it is sometimes difficult to come to the doctor that often. It looks like your blood pressure is still elevated today. What's your blood pressure been at home?"

Mr. Bernard shifts his weight in the chair, and says, "I'm not sure, Doc. We've been adding medications and increasing medications, and I'm just not sure they're working. Is there something else we can do?" Bri'elle identifies an opportunity to educate the patient. She launches into a soliloquy about lifestyle changes (he is built for hypertension, being slightly obese with a round figure), weight loss, and alcohol and sodium intake effects on elevated blood pressure. She offers several bits of advice on how to decrease caloric intake by reducing portion size, stresses the importance of minimal to moderate alcohol consumption, and also identifies examples of high-salt foods. Mr. Bernard listens attentively and nods frequently. Bri'elle asks if he has any questions or any other concerns today. He replies that he does not, and she exits the room.

In the hallway, she catches up with her attending physician, Robert, and they huddle with the clinic nurse, Nancy Perez. Bri'elle relates her encounter with Mr. Bernard, and Robert nods knowingly. Nancy says, "He's been here twice in the past three months for blood pressure checks, and each time I have told him about losing weight and about decreasing his alcohol and salt intake. I have looked at our panel data and have identified that about 20% of our patients are over the goal of 140/90. I wonder if there is a system change that we can make to meet our patients' needs in a more effective manner?"

Nancy shares the many reasons for why blood pressure may remain high for some of their panel patients. "It may be due to their diet, adherence with taking the medications as prescribed, or stress." Robert asks Nancy and Bri'elle, "Did either of you ask him whether he is taking all his medications as prescribed?" Bri'elle replies sheepishly, "I never got around to it; I was so intent on making sure I gave him the counseling that I thought he needed." "Let's go back in," Robert says, "and see him together. I wonder whether he's been taking all the meds and what factors might be contributing to his lifestyle choices." Meanwhile, Nancy continues to think about the 20% of their patients whose hypertension is not controlled and starts thinking about ways the clinic might partner with them in better blood pressure management.

# The Complexity of Systems Changes

It may seem odd to start a chapter on systems change by describing an individual patient encounter. For most of this book, we have focused the aims, the process modeling, and the measurement on *systems of care* for populations of patients. So why do we now switch to a story of an individual patient to start the discussion of change? Recall the description of the levels of the health care system in Chapter 4, with the target diagram (*see* Figure 4-5 on page 64). It shows that at the center of every system in health care is the patient, in relation to his or her own self-care system. The frustration in this chapter's opening vignette is evident—the frustration of the medical student, the nurse, the physician, and the patient. We sometimes act as if the patient exists in isolation and that the changes in lifestyle and medication regimen we recommend will occur automatically when a patient exits the office. We "pull the lever" of adding a medication and expect an equal and simple reaction on the other end of the "machine"—in the life of the patient and in his or her physiology.

In this case, the clinical team expected a lowering of Mr. Bernard's blood pressure. When we do not get the response we expect (for example, the blood pressure is still elevated, the patient's weight has increased a few pounds), we may be tempted to place the blame on the patient by saying that the patient is noncompliant with our recommendations. This "one cause/one effect" relationship is a linear cause-and-effect sequence:

**Patient with hypertension + Medication**
**= Patient with lower blood pressure from medication**
**or**
**Patient with hypertension + Education**
**= Patient with lower blood pressure from increased knowledge**

Although sometimes the relationship plays out in this aligned, sequential linear model, systems—even patient self-care systems—are usually not that simple. In fact, the issue may be due to gaps in the system of care.

*Nancy, Robert, and Bri'elle sit down and start to brainstorm potential ways the system can better support patients like*

*Mr. Bernard in their self-management efforts. They talk about issues of health literacy, cognitive function, side effects of medications, and patients' understanding of their medications prior to leaving the clinic. Nancy agrees to ask several patients about their medications the next day.*

*She reports back to the group that 50% of the 20 patients she talked with were unsure about the purpose of their medications, 25% were confused about what medications to take at the time of the clinic discharge, and 40% did not have a reminder system in place to ensure that they took their medications. Forty percent of the patients reported that the clinic's after-visit summary was not helpful.*

## Completing the Model for Improvement

This chapter completes the explanation of the Model for Improvement that started in Chapter 1 (*see* Figure 7-1, right).[1] Sometimes improvement work starts when we make changes to a system without the foundational work of a clear aim, understanding of the processes, and identification of measures. Chapters 3 and 4 cover identifying an aim for improvement and modeling the process ("What are we trying to accomplish?"), and Chapters 5 and 6 explore measurement for improvement ("How will we know that a change is an improvement?"). We now turn our attention to making changes with patients to improve care.

### The two-part final stage of the Model for Improvement

The final stage of the Model for Improvement has two parts: (1) "What change can we make that will result in improvement?" and (2) the Plan–Do–Study–Act (PDSA) cycle. This two-step final stage allows an improvement team to first generate a list of possible changes that might be helpful (that is, brainstorm) and then to make small tests of these changes, using PDSA cycles. Remaining faithful to the rigors of the Model for Improvement will confirm the aphorism that "all improvement requires change, but not all change leads to improvement."[2]

### The evidence-based improvement formula applied to changes in a system

In Chapter 1 we introduced the evidence-based improvement formula (*see* Figure 1-3 on page 15).[3] This formula describes how the evidence that is derived from research (effectiveness of care) is combined with the knowledge of systems and processes to achieve improved patient outcomes. In Chapter 1 we described the main components of this formula. In Chapter 3 we discussed

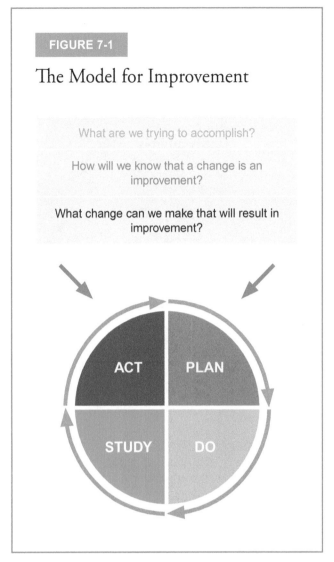

Source: Adapted from Langley GJ, et al. *The Improvement Guide: A Practical Approach to Enhancing Organizational Performance*, 2nd ed. San Francisco: Jossey-Bass, 2009. Printed with permission.

other potential areas to consider for improvement, such as the safety of the care we deliver, the efficiency of the delivery of care, and ensuring that care is equitable. We have modified the evidence-based improvement formula (*see* Figure 7-2 on the next page) to emphasize these broader opportunities for improvement. In other words, we have the potential to improve the quality of care in many ways related to the Institute of Medicine quality domains.[4] In addition, we note here that the plus sign (+) and the arrow (→) play a key role when considering changes in a system. The + is an indication of how the improvement opportunities and the local setting or particular context are brought together. This is not a haphazard connection but requires a plan of change and a plan for linking the

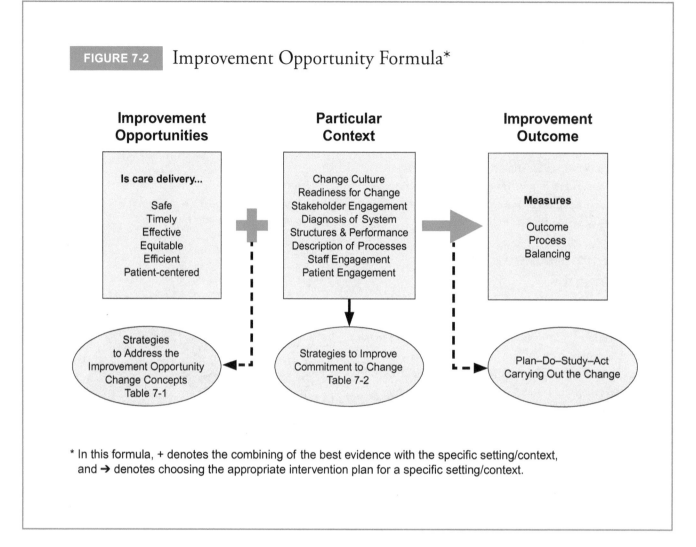

**FIGURE 7-2** Improvement Opportunity Formula*

**Improvement Opportunities**

Is care delivery...

Safe
Timely
Effective
Equitable
Efficient
Patient-centered

Strategies
to Address the
Improvement Opportunity
Change Concepts
Table 7-1

**Particular Context**

Change Culture
Readiness for Change
Stakeholder Engagement
Diagnosis of System
Structures & Performance
Description of Processes
Staff Engagement
Patient Engagement

Strategies to Improve
Commitment to Change
Table 7-2

**Improvement Outcome**

Measures

Outcome
Process
Balancing

Plan–Do–Study–Act
Carrying Out the Change

\* In this formula, + denotes the combining of the best evidence with the specific setting/context, and ➔ denotes choosing the appropriate intervention plan for a specific setting/context.

improvement intervention to the local practice. (Further strategies to address this will be described later in the chapter.) The ➔ refers to executing and managing the plan in the local setting. Carrying out the plan involves knowing the resources that are available to make it happen. The change must connect to the ways things work in a particular setting. It is at this step that the PDSA cycle will be used to test each change.

The improvement opportunity formula in Figure 7-2 helps us appreciate the complexity of change in health care systems, which rarely react in a linear fashion. Instead, health care reacts in an adaptive manner, as a complex adaptive system. A *complex adaptive system* (CAS) is defined as "a collection of individual agents that have the freedom to act in ways that are not always predictable and whose actions are interconnected such that one agent's actions changes the context for the other agents."[5 (pp. 312–313)] Each agent's actions influence the *context* of the system,

so understanding the context, culture, and processes of care are vital to successful change in a CAS. Other examples of CASs are biologic (like an ant colony) and economic (like the stock market).

As a CAS is perturbed by change, the system achieves a new steady state. This holds true for single-celled organisms and also for large health care organizations. The tension, uncertainty, and anxiety that come with change are healthy elements in complex systems to achieve greater performance. There are eight principal properties of CASs that enable us to identify the components and interactions within the system. See the appendix for the complete list of the CAS properties and an example that highlights the components.

So why is understanding the complexity of systems important for making changes in a health care setting? Complexity theory shifts our thinking from systems as mechanical, linear interactions to nonlinear, emergent, and embedded sets of interconnected, adaptable elements. There will be times when a health care system (for example, private-practice office, unit in a hospital, nursing department) will want to "install," "implement," or "roll out" a new process. These words should be concerning because they signal an assumption that change is mechanical. We pull a lever (have training, send a memo), "install" a change, and the system is better. When we hear these words from those who intend to make changes in health care, we need to be wary of their underlying assumptions about the system.

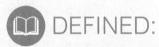 DEFINED:

### Complex Adaptive System (CAS)

A *complex adaptive system (CAS)* is a collection of individual agents that have the freedom to act in ways that are not always predictable and whose actions are interconnected such that one agent's actions changes the context for the other agents.

*After reviewing the patient data with Robert and Bri'elle, Nancy shares an idea that might address the quality gap. She provides a website link to the teach-back method.[6] The website explains that the teach-back method is a way of checking understanding by having patients state in their own words what they need to manage their own health. The teach-back method is a way to confirm that your explanation to the patient is understood. Nancy suggests that the routine use of teach-back in the clinic might be a way to ensure that patients understand their medications before leaving. Robert wonders if patients would be receptive to adding this to the visit. The team decides to ask a small group of patients to get their feedback, and the patients think this approach would be helpful. Now the work to make the change begins, and the team must consider the clinic as a CAS.*

*To better understand the clinic as a CAS, Robert, Nancy, and Bri'elle start by recruiting a patient with hypertension to become a part of their quality improvement team. Together they reflect on the concepts of a CAS to anticipate ways to ensure a smooth testing of the teach-back method in the clinic visits. The team considers the nonlinear property of CASs and anticipates that small changes may have a large effect and that it is possible that large changes may have a small effect.*

*Team members also are aware that they must consider culture and context to identify underlying elements that may influence the functioning of the system. They also anticipate that a proposed change to the current system may cause anxiety, tension, and uncertainty among staff. The properties of the CAS may seem overwhelming, but the team is up for the challenge.*

## Managing Changes in a System

Now that you have been introduced to how systems respond to change, how do you start managing these changes? There are multiple theories of managing change; in fact, entire books have been written on managing change in organizations. Here we present a scenario about reducing falls and injuries due to falls on a hospital unit. We use this scenario to describe the basic elements of change theory, introduce one technique to identify possible changes based on the process diagram, and discuss the PDSA cycles. We'll return to the hypertension team's work later in the chapter.

*Yinzhi Chen, a registered nurse who also holds a doctoral degree, has been the chief nursing officer at the academic Bayside Medical Center (BMC) for the past three years. She is frequently amazed at the size and complexity of BMC. In addition to undergraduate nursing, nurse practitioner, and nurse anesthetist students who fall under her responsibility, there are resident physicians, medical students, pharmacy students and interns, and students from respiratory, physical, and occupational therapy. The educational focus of BMC makes it an exciting (and challenging) organization at which to work.*

*Today Yinzhi is not focused on the teaching mission but is instead consumed by some rather troubling information. The patient fall rate at BMC has been high and steady for several years. Yinzhi spent many years as a medical/surgical nurse, and she knows that a patient fall can cause serious injury and is an adverse outcome for that patient. A patient who falls and has a serious injury such as a hip fracture can have a one-year mortality rate near 33%.[7] As the chief nursing officer, she realizes that there is no simple solution. She'll need to enlist a team of individuals from many professions to solve this problem. She reviews the data from different units and ponders some possible actions. Perhaps a day-long education event about patients' risk of falling? She could start with the lowest-performing ward; it can only go up. Perhaps she could bring in a consultant team to recommend some changes?*

*Yinzhi decides to confer with Gerry Rogale, the medical chief of staff. He was surprised to see the high rate of falls on so many of the wards. The medicine ward has the poorest performance in the hospital, but Yinzhi and Gerry decide against starting there. The medicine ward has been under some stress due to the retirement of the long-term chief of medicine two months ago and now have an interim chief in place. The Physical Medicine and Rehabilitation (PM&R) Unit might be a possibility. Yinzhi and Gerry have had a good working relationship with this group. The PM&R fall rate is a little below the hospital average, and there are strong leaders in the unit in nursing, medicine, and physical therapy. This is a group that could tackle the problem of patient falls and identify some changes that might work for the entire organization. Yinzhi and Gerry agree that this is a reasonable place to start and decide to charge a team to lower the rate of falls on the BMC PM&R unit.*

## Patterns of Responses to Change/Innovation

After Yinzhi and Gerry decided to create a quality improvement project to reduce falls, their next decision was where to start. They did not "roll out" a program for the entire hospital but instead focused on identifying a unit that would be best suited to work on the problem. In his theory of "diffusion of innovations," Everett Rogers developed a classification for considering how change is adopted and disseminated within a system.[8] Choosing the right starting place for change depends on identifying the characteristics of the people and system that will be changed.

*Classifying the responders.* Rogers identified five different patterns of responses to innovation or change (*see* Figure 7-3 on page 115). The classification of responders is based on these patterns:

- **Group 1—Innovators:** Change often starts with innovators. The innovators are the smallest subgroup and often are the creative and passionate individuals.
- **Group 2—Early adopters:** The next group is the early adopters, who are often respected opinion leaders within the system and are role models for others. As shown in Figure 7-3, early adopters are positioned on the initial upslope of accepting and incorporating a change. These individuals (or the systems in which they work) are willing to try changes and work out the bugs to identify what works and what does not work. Yinzhi and Gerry recognize that the PM&R unit is an early adopter unit. With strong leadership in medicine, nursing, and physical therapy, this unit likely is a good place to try new ideas and work out how best to address the patient falls problem.

- **Group 3—Early majority:** The next type of responders is the early majority, who represent a critical stage for widespread acceptance of a change. This is the group that, when successfully adopting a change, is able to bring the change to the peak rate of acceptance. The early majority considers the pros and cons of the change and will discuss the changes with others to get a feel for the situation. When the early majority adopts a change, more generalized acceptance likely will follow.
- **Group 4—Late majority:** The fourth innovation responder category is the late majority. Those in this group often require a bit of friendly peer pressure to take up an innovation.
- **Group 5—Laggards:** The laggards are the final group. Although this term may seem pejorative, the laggards perform an important cross-checking role. They may be suspicious of a new idea and often look to the past instead of the future. For laggards, resistance to an innovation is rational because they must be certain that important things they value about the current state of affairs will not be lost in the new way of operating.

These response patterns regarding the diffusion of innovations are not intended to be a series of boxes in which to place individuals, clinical units, or microsystems. In reality, each person has times when he or she is an innovator, part of the early majority, or a laggard. Someone who is an innovator in one instance might be a laggard in another. Similarly, an ambulatory pediatric practice might be an innovator in using new computer technology but a laggard in adopting a new form for documenting patient home instructions. The important message from Figure 7-3 is that the diffusion of change is a process that occurs across a continuum. Simply offering a change and hoping that it will be taken up and spread throughout the system is not an effective strategy. Rogers's observations about the different patterns of response to new ideas can help identify where and with whom to develop and carry out new ideas.

Let's return to the scenario to examine the next steps.

*The leaders on the PM&R unit charge an interprofessional team to lead the falls improvement project. The team consists of five members: Jaime Fernandez, one of the floor nurses; Christine Sun, the chief resident in PM&R; Peter Hampton, a physical therapist; Sam Jones, a patient recently discharged from the unit, and Corinna Ajit, the unit pharmacist. This month, they are joined by Amira Salat, a final-semester nursing student who is interested in PM&R. She is doing a clinical rotation on the ward. The team obtains the patient falls data from Yinzhi. The team members at first don't*

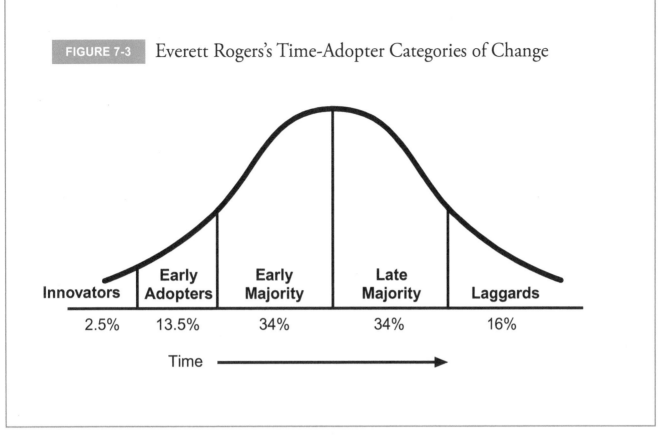

**FIGURE 7-3**    Everett Rogers's Time-Adopter Categories of Change

| Innovators | Early Adopters | Early Majority | Late Majority | Laggards |
|:---:|:---:|:---:|:---:|:---:|
| 2.5% | 13.5% | 34% | 34% | 16% |

Time ⟶

Source: Adapted from Rogers EM. *Diffusion of Innovations*, 4th ed. New York: Free Press, 1995.

understand why their unit was chosen to be the first to work on the falls initiative. The data win them over. They are surprised to see that the rate of falls (adjusted for the number of bed-days of care per month) has been stable, with a rather high average, for the past 24 months (see Figure 7-4 on page 116). The rate shows only common-cause variation. (See Chapter 6 for information about common-cause variation.) If the system on the PM&R unit continues as is, the unit can expect (or predict) a monthly fall rate between 1.1 (lower control limit) and 12.4 (upper control limit). Because this is a rehabilitation unit that focuses on patient mobility and function, the team is disappointed with these results. The team thought the unit was doing better than this.

Sam is excited to be part of the improvement team because when he was a patient on the unit he was frustrated with some of the care he received. He learned about improvement as a manager of quality in a local manufacturing company. The PM&R unit team agrees on an aim: "Reduce the fall rate on the BMC PM&R unit by 50% over the next nine months." The team members recognize the need to have a common process diagram to guide their discussions. Amira and Sam agree to follow a few patients through the care

process on the ward and create a deployment flowchart. They share their efforts with the team at the meeting the following week (see Figure 7-5 on page 117).

## Identifying Possible Changes Using Change Concepts

In Chapter 4 we discussed the importance of understanding the context and the processes of care. Creating a process model helps us to develop a common representation of a process and allows a team to identify possible changes to make. The list of possible changes often comes from best practices or from individuals who are part of the process (including the patients and families) and have ideas about how it can be improved. Whatever it chooses, a team cannot be sure of success until the change is tested and the team evaluates the reaction of the system.

Beyond best practices and personal experience within the system, change concepts can help a team use a process diagram to identify ways to improve the system. *Change concepts* are general principles that can be applied to any clinical process. Langley et al. listed 72 change concepts

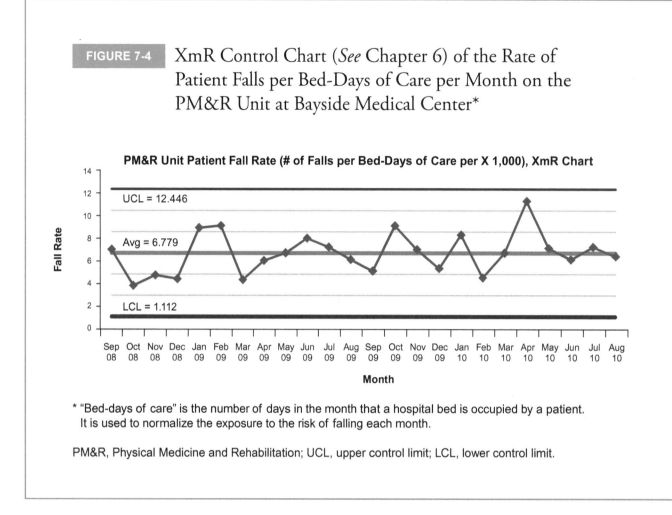

**FIGURE 7-4** XmR Control Chart (*See* Chapter 6) of the Rate of Patient Falls per Bed-Days of Care per Month on the PM&R Unit at Bayside Medical Center*

**PM&R Unit Patient Fall Rate (# of Falls per Bed-Days of Care per X 1,000), XmR Chart**

UCL = 12.446

Avg = 6.779

LCL = 1.112

Fall Rate

Sep 08, Oct 08, Nov 08, Dec 08, Jan 09, Feb 09, Mar 09, Apr 09, May 09, Jun 09, Jul 09, Aug 09, Sep 09, Oct 09, Nov 09, Dec 09, Jan 10, Feb 10, Mar 10, Apr 10, May 10, Jun 10, Jul 10, Aug 10

**Month**

\* "Bed-days of care" is the number of days in the month that a hospital bed is occupied by a patient. It is used to normalize the exposure to the risk of falling each month.

PM&R, Physical Medicine and Rehabilitation; UCL, upper control limit; LCL, lower control limit.

from their work improving many different types of systems.[1] Nelson et al.[9] winnowed down these 72 general change concepts to 10 that are most applicable to health care (*see* Table 7-1 on page 118 and Figure 7-6 on page 120).

A *change concept* "is a general notion or approach to change found to be useful in developing specific ideas for changes that lead to improvement."[1(p. 357)] These generic concepts can clarify a team's thinking about where (and how) in a process a change should occur. In some cases, the 10 change concepts merely put names to changes that a team has already identified. If an improvement team has clear and reasonable ideas about where the process needs to change, the change can start there. A team can use the change concepts as a complement to its thinking when it is stalled or when it needs a different approach. The change concepts make a sort of toolbox the team can open when it needs to think differently about the process. For example, change concept 4 in Figure 7-6 is to "eliminate a step," and change concept 10 is to "listen to customers (patients, families,

staff)." A process flow diagram, like the one shown in Figure 7-5, often identifies unnecessary and repetitive steps in a process; however, it may be difficult in a process diagram to identify the opportunity to create changes because a team does not always get feedback from customers. For example, the BMC PM&R unit had been using soft wrist restraints for patients who developed acute delirium while on the unit. These restraints can be effective for keeping a patient safe for a short period of time, but families were troubled by seeing the restraints. This important feedback from families helped the team consider alternatives to restraints to keep patients safe.

Change concepts related to the process of care are important, but there are other change concepts that can be considered beyond the process focus. The field of implementation science has generated a list of evidence-based change concepts or strategies to enhance the adoption, implementation, and sustainability of a change in clinical practice.[10,11] The Expert Recommendations for

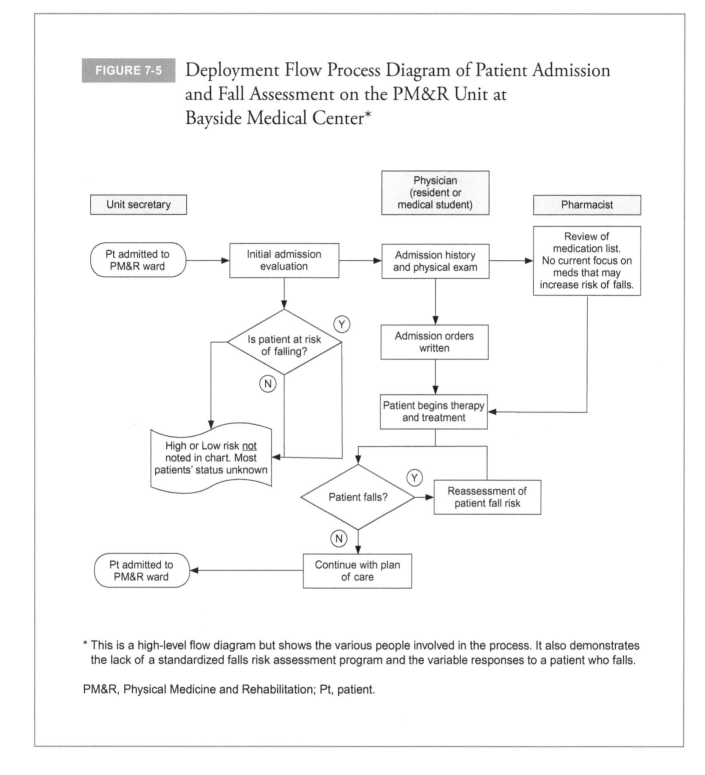

**FIGURE 7-5**  Deployment Flow Process Diagram of Patient Admission and Fall Assessment on the PM&R Unit at Bayside Medical Center*

* This is a high-level flow diagram but shows the various people involved in the process. It also demonstrates the lack of a standardized falls risk assessment program and the variable responses to a patient who falls.

PM&R, Physical Medicine and Rehabilitation; Pt, patient.

Implementation Change (ERIC) project outlines terms and definitions for 73 discrete implementation strategies that have been described in the health care literature.[10] The strategies are grouped into nine categories and are (a) evaluative and iterative strategies such as audit and feedback, (b) interactive assistance strategies such as facilitation or coaching, (c) strategies for adapting and tailoring implementation to local context such as with tailored strategy selection, (d) strategies for developing stakeholder interrelationships such as with the use of champions and coalition building, (e) training and education strategies, (f) strategies for supporting clinicians/educators, (g) engagement strategies for consumers/students, (h) financial strategies, and (i) strategies for

| Concept Number | Change Concept Name | Description | Example* |
|---|---|---|---|
| **TABLE 7-1** | | **Description and Examples of Change Concepts That Can Be Used to Improve Any Clinical Process** | |
| 1 | Modify input | The process has a starting point, and this starting point can be changed. | Screen patients for risk of falling at admission to the unit. |
| 2 | Combine steps | The team should combine steps in the process where time and resources can be saved. | Because assessment is completed at admission, falls risk notation ("falling star") is completed up front rather than several days into a patient's admission. |
| 3 | Eliminate failures at handoffs | Handoffs require clear, consistent, and reliable transfer of information. | At nursing sign-out, make the falls risk score one of the vital signs. |
| 4 | Eliminate a step | The team should identify steps in a process that add no value to the system. | Physical therapists do not need to redo falls assessment. Initial nursing assessment includes adequate information for all professionals. |
| 5 | Reorder the sequence of steps | Perhaps prioritizing steps in a different way would help the work flow. | Toileting often occurs after distributing meds. Distributing meds can take a long time, so move toileting to before giving meds. |
| 6 | Smooth the work flow in a step | The demand for services causes a large bolus in the number of patients and disrupts the overall flow. | The workup and documentation of possible injuries in a patient who falls is not standardized. |
| 7 | Replace with a better value step | Sometimes a step in a process is just not working well and needs to be completely replaced. | Patients are usually randomly assigned to rooms on the ward. Place patients at high risk of falls close to the nurses' station. |
| 8 | From knowledge of outcome, redesign process | Outcome and process measures create a powerful impetus for change and can also direct the team to certain specific changes. | Further analysis of the fall rate data shows that patients with a history of stroke have a higher rate of falls. |

*See Figure 7-6 on page 120.

| TABLE 7-1 | Description and Examples of Change Concepts That Can Be Used to Improve Any Clinical Process *(continued)* | | |
|---|---|---|---|
| **Concept Number** | **Change Concept Name** | **Description** | **Example*** |
| 9 | Do tasks in parallel with the main process | Improvements in time and costs can be made by recognition that some tasks can be completed at the same time rather than in sequence. | Falls risk assessment can occur with initial nursing intake. |
| 10 | Listen to customers (patients, families, staff) | Input about our processes from the users of our services can often provide significant insight into how to improve what we do. | Families express concern about the use of restraints when patients have acute delirium. Identify alternative ways of preventing falls rather than restraints. |

**Source:** Adapted from Nelson EC, Batalden PB, Lazar JS, editors. *Practice-Based Learning and Improvement: A Clinical Improvement Action Guide*, 2nd ed. Oak Brook, IL: Joint Commission Resources, 2007.

*See Figure 7-6 on page 120.

changing the infrastructure.[12] See the appendix for more detail and use of some of these strategies.

Generating a list of possible change strategies answers the third question in the Model for Improvement: What change can we make that will result in improvement? (*See* Figure 7-1 on page 111.) The team is now ready to try some of these changes.

*Amira's and Sam's work on the process diagram is immensely helpful to the team. The team members immediately recognize that there is no consistent way to identify patients at high risk of falling (see Figure 7-5). Reducing falls is going to be nearly impossible if the team cannot identify the patients who are at high risk. The team decides to test a fall risk–assessment tool. Amira will help Jaime with this tool for the next few patients admitted to the unit. They use the PDSA approach (introduced in Chapter 1) to guide their work (see Figure 7-1):*

*PDSA 1*
**Plan**—*Jaime, the floor nurse, will use a standard fall risk–assessment tool on the next three patients admitted to him on the PM&R unit.*

**Do**—*Jaime administers the fall risk–assessment tool to Mrs. Perez, a 78-year-old woman who is recovering from a left cerebral stroke; Mr. Browne, a 68-year-old man who had a hip replacement; and Ms. Nichols, a 36-year-old woman who had shoulder surgery. Amira observes each trial and times the administration of the instrument. She identifies Mrs. Perez and Mr. Browne as being at high risk for falling, but determines Ms. Nichols is not.*

**Study**—*Jaime and Amira debrief with the improvement team. Although the fall risk assessment seems to be accurate in that it identifies patients at high risk, it is cumbersome to administer. It took Jaime an average of 4 minutes and 23 seconds for each patient. In addition, some of the information on the form is already collected as part of the intake information on the ward.*

**Act**—*Conducting a fall risk assessment is important, but the current form is too cumbersome to use in addition to completing other duties.*

*Amira identifies a short form from the material that Peter the physical therapist brought back from a recent conference. The*

Example of 10 Change Concepts Applied to Any Process*

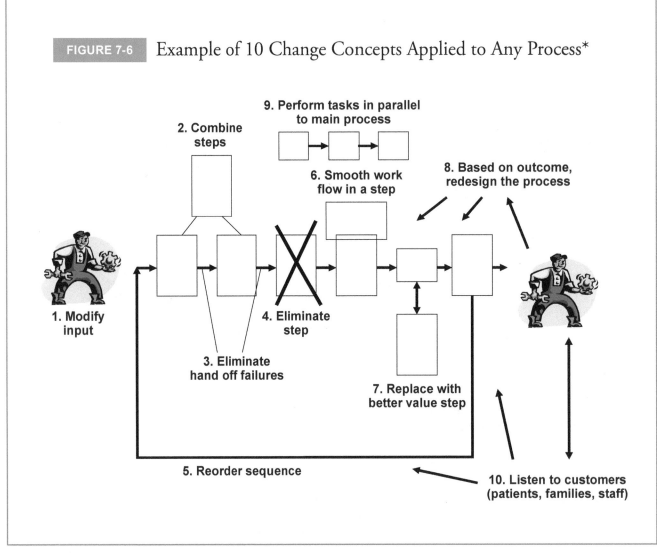

Users might present the 10 change concepts as a visual, such as the flow diagram in this figure.
* See Table 7-1 on pages118–119 and the text for more details.

**Source:** Adapted from Nelson EC, Batalden PB, Lazar JS, editors. *Practice-Based Learning and Improvement: A Clinical Improvement Action Guide*, 2nd ed. Oak Brook, IL: Joint Commission Resources, 2007.

*short form of the fall risk–assessment tool works much better than the old form. Jaime finds it easy to administer, it provides valuable information, and Amira scores the administration time at just under 40 seconds, which is acceptable to both nurses and patients.*

*Now that they can reliably identify patients at high risk, the team tries several other interventions to decrease the rate of falls. It moves high-risk patients closer to the nurses' station and pilot tests bed alarms and chair alarms. It also identifies each high-risk patient with a "falling star" on his or her*

*doorpost and purchases some low beds for very high-risk patients. Table 7-2 on page 121 provides a complete list of changes the team tried.*

*After six months of work and 12 different PDSA cycles, the team is pleased to see that the fall rate has dropped below the lower control limit, indicating special-cause variation (see Figure 7-7 on page 122). The team is encouraged by this signal in the data that reflects the work done. The unit now has a reliable fall risk–assessment tool and evidence-based interventions that prevent patient falls.*

*The team meets with Yinzhi and Gerry to discuss its progress. Team members are excited about the results and are anxious to spread the interventions to other units in the hospital. Figure 7-7 on page 122 shows the updated XmR chart, with a few months of fall rates under the mean of 6.5 and a special cause represented in the most recent data point. The arrows indicate the tested changes. Dark arrows indicate changes that were successful and maintained, and lighter arrows are changes that were not successful and, therefore, not continued.*

## Using the PDSA Cycles to Test and Assess Changes

As introduced in Chapter 1, we use the Model for Improvement and PDSA cycles to test changes in a system (*see* Figure 7-8 on page 123). The PDSA cycle is intended to test small changes, but sometimes we apply it to large-scale changes or to planned changes that have not been completed. For example, we might state that the implementation of a new electronic health record (EHR) uses PDSA cycles in the following way:

| | |
|---|---|
| **Plan** | Implement a new EHR. |
| **Do** | Get the new EHR installed. |
| **Study** | Assess the uptake and use of the new EHR. |
| **Act** | Improve the use of the new EHR, based on preliminary findings. |

This example, however, demonstrates a common misconception and misuse of PDSA cycles. PDSA cycles work best when applied to testing small changes in a system. It is generally not appropriate for testing the rollout of a new massive change effort. Large-scale change efforts use a different methodology, such as an organizationwide strategic plan. We use a PDSA cycle to test one change with a few patients in one setting on a small scale. This approach may feel too small to make a difference, but the goal is to build knowledge about the process step-by-step. The improvement team rarely stops at just one PDSA cycle. Jaime and Amira performed the first PDSA cycle for the BMC PM&R falls team by trying an assessment tool on three patients. This test provided a wealth of information for the team. The team recognized that the tool was effective but cumbersome to administer. If falls assessment were to become a routine part of the admission process, a faster, more reliable form would be needed.

The four phases of the PDSA cycle are as follows (*see* Figure 7-8):

- **Plan:** The team starts in the "Plan" phase, in which team members state the goal of the test of change. This is different from the overall aim of the improvement

project (as discussed in Chapter 3) because PDSA plans are very focused and directed at the immediate test of change. The Plan phase also encourages the team to create a hypothesis about what will happen when it tries this change. Finally, the Plan phase specifies who will do what, and where and when this will occur.

- **Do:** Carrying out the test and documenting observations about the test occur in the "Do" phase. The evaluation of the Do phase may be quantitative, but often with small tests of change a qualitative analysis is equally effective to determine what occurred.

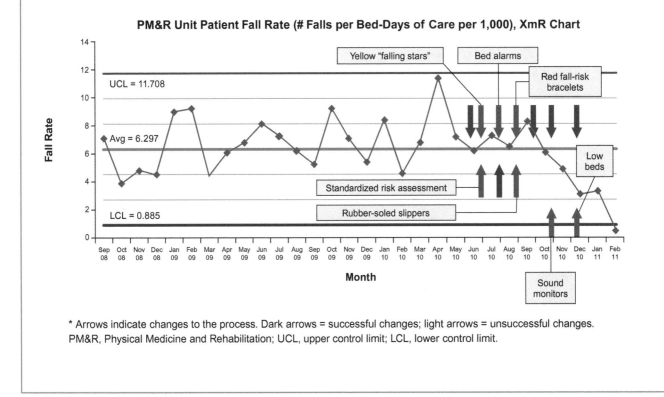

**FIGURE 7-7** Updated and Annotated XmR Chart of the Fall Rate for the PM&R Unit at Bayside Medical Center*

PM&R Unit Patient Fall Rate (# Falls per Bed-Days of Care per 1,000), XmR Chart

Yellow "falling stars"

Bed alarms

Red fall-risk bracelets

UCL = 11.708

Avg = 6.297

Standardized risk assessment

Low beds

Rubber-soled slippers

LCL = 0.885

Fall Rate

Sep 08 · Oct 08 · Nov 08 · Dec 08 · Jan 09 · Feb 09 · Mar 09 · Apr 09 · May 09 · Jun 09 · Jul 09 · Aug 09 · Sep 09 · Oct 09 · Nov 09 · Dec 09 · Jan 10 · Feb 10 · Mar 10 · Apr 10 · May 10 · Jun 10 · Jul 10 · Aug 10 · Sep 10 · Oct 10 · Nov 10 · Dec 10 · Jan 11 · Feb 11

Month

Sound monitors

* Arrows indicate changes to the process. Dark arrows = successful changes; light arrows = unsuccessful changes.
PM&R, Physical Medicine and Rehabilitation; UCL, upper control limit; LCL, lower control limit.

- **Study:** In the "Study" phase the team will perform a complete analysis of the data. Here team members compare the measured outcome against the predicted outcome, and then summarize.

- **Act:** The "Act" phase consists of determining the consequences of the change. What will be the objective for the next PDSA cycle? The Act phase from one PDSA cycle flows into the Plan phase of the subsequent cycle.

*Assessing successive PDSA cycles.* PDSA cycles are iterative and build upon one another. Figure 7-9 on page 124 shows an example of successive PDSA cycles progressing "uphill" as the improvement in the system increases over time. Each PDSA cycle generates new knowledge about the system as tests are tried. Each successive PDSA cycle requires an increase in complexity as we gather knowledge about the system. It is never intended that one PDSA cycle will achieve the aim stated at the outset. Rather, each PDSA

cycle is a small experiment that advances the team's knowledge about the system. Recall that systems behave in complex, adaptive ways, and it is difficult to predict exactly how the system will respond. Figure 7-9 shows a tidy progression of PDSAs as the system improves. In the complexity of real changes in a system, there are often incomplete PDSAs, irregular PDSAs, and barriers that emerge. Figure 7-10 on page 125 provides a more realistic depiction of how PDSAs progress over time.[13]

Using PDSAs is often messy and can be difficult . . . this is OK, as the goal is to accumulate knowledge and insight about the system as changes are made.

Each PDSA cycle allows the team to assess how the system responds to changes. The team will maintain and amplify successful changes and discard unsuccessful changes. The falls team will record those changes tried, those maintained, and those discontinued.

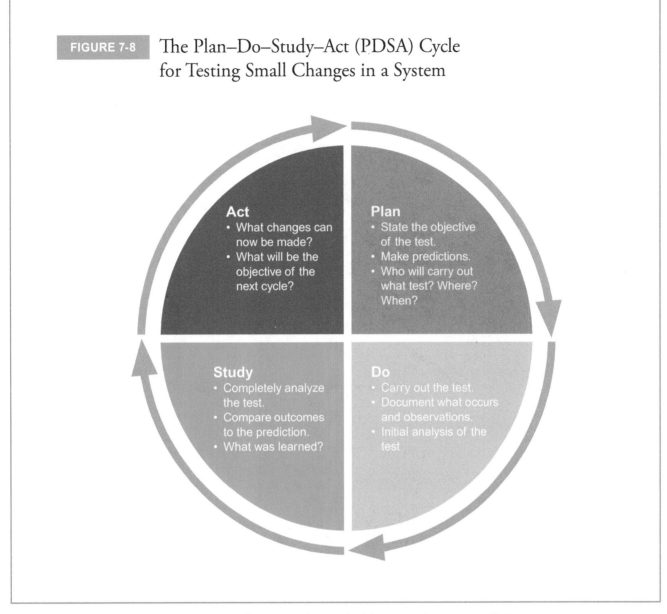

**FIGURE 7-8** The Plan–Do–Study–Act (PDSA) Cycle for Testing Small Changes in a System

The last step in the Model for Improvement, PDSA Cycles, provides a methodology to test improvement efforts.

**Source:** Langley GJ, et al. *The Improvement Guide: A Practical Approach to Enhancing Organizational Performance*, 2nd ed. San Francisco: Jossey-Bass, 2009. Printed with permission.

*Monitoring and tracking PDSA cycles.* The most successful users of PDSA cycles are those who monitor and track the cycles in an organized fashion. This is akin to maintaining a lab notebook in laboratory research. As the PDSA cycles grow in number, the team may forget what Cycles 1, 2, and 3 contained because each cycle grows on the previous one. By the time the team gets to Cycle 8 (or 23 or 37), team members may not recall what occurred in the early cycles. Having a lab notebook to keep track of the tests of change is a convenient way to monitor the changes they have tried.

## Embedding knowledge gained from the Model for Improvement into a system

After a team has identified and studied effective interventions in a system with rapid-cycle PDSA cycles, how can these changes be embedded in a system? What is to prevent these good practices that improved outcomes from decaying over time? Sustaining changes in a system requires at least two elements: (1) interventions that are hardwired into the system and (2) regular review of process and outcome measures. Both require the attention of leaders (*see* Chapter 8 for more on sustaining change).

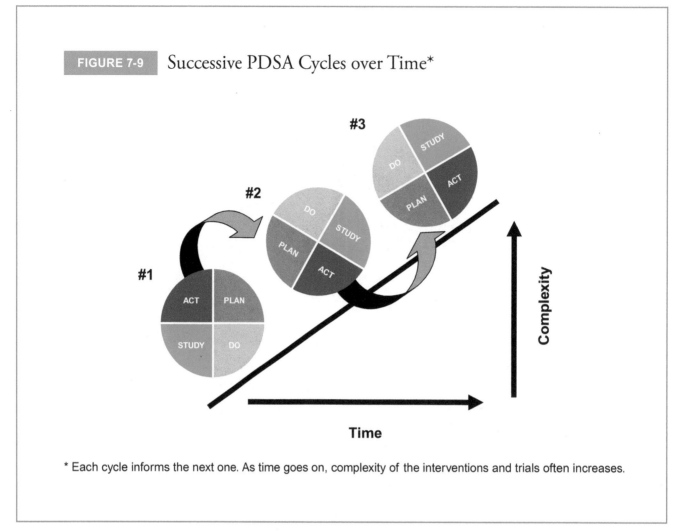

**FIGURE 7-9**   Successive PDSA Cycles over Time*

#3

#2

#1

Complexity

Time

\* Each cycle informs the next one. As time goes on, complexity of the interventions and trials often increases.

**Source:** Adapted from Nelson EC, Batalden PB, Lazar JS, editors. *Practice-Based Learning and Improvement: A Clinical Improvement Action Guide*, 2nd ed. Oak Brook, IL: Joint Commission Resources, 2007.

In this chapter's example, Amira and Jaime implemented a tool through several PDSA cycles for fall risk stratification of new admissions. Making this a lasting part of the work on the PM&R unit will require that the new form be integrated into the admission routine for all nurses. Knowledge of the usual process of admission (*see* Figure 7-5, page 117) will help, as will support from the leadership on the unit. Without the regular evaluation of measures (*see* Figure 7-7, page 122), it will be nearly impossible for a team to assess the lasting effectiveness and sustainability of the change. PDSA cycles encourage rigor and also demand humility from the improvement team. The rigor comes from the discipline of using a standard, focused methodology for making change that requires iterative hypothesis generation coupled with measurement of outcomes. The humility comes with the recognition and realization that complex systems react in often

unpredictable, adaptive ways. With hypothesis generation, careful measurement, and synthesis of outcomes, a team can determine whether the changes it tries truly lead to improvements.

To improve the rate of patient falls at Bayside Medical Center, Yinzhi and Gerry used principles from Rogers's diffusion of innovations classification. They used change concepts that included improvement team champions and provided education and support the staff needed (including data) to identify and test a series of changes over time. The team learned which changes worked in its setting by tracking the results over time. During the team's improvement journey, there were many barriers to change. These barriers to change required new interventions to move the improvement work forward.

**FIGURE 7-10** Revised Model of Successive PDSAs with Barriers, Background Interference, and Incomplete Cycles

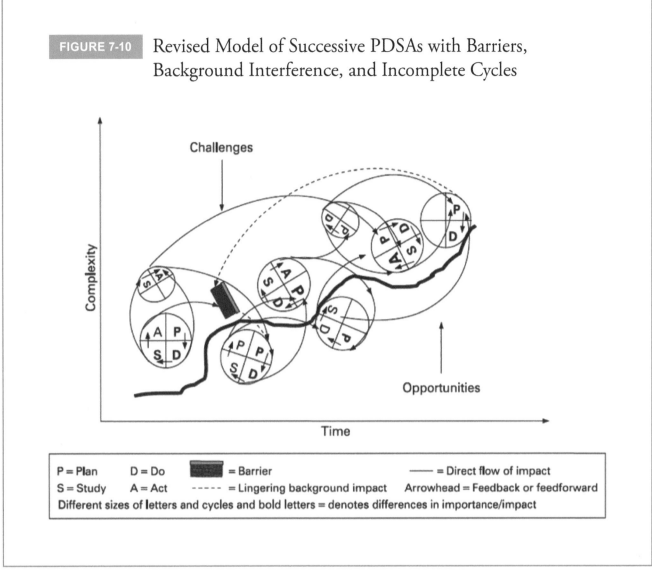

**Source:** Tomolo A, Lawrence R, Aron D. A case study of translating the ACGME practice-based learning and improvement requirements into reality: systems quality improvement projects as the key component to a comprehensive curriculum. *Postgrad Med J* 2009; 85:530–7. Reprinted with permission from BMJ Publishing Group Limited.

## Barriers to Change

Despite the best planning and targeting of changes, barriers to change are common. Change disrupts the patterns and processes that are in place, so pushback is to be expected. Barriers to change often feel immense and, perhaps, insurmountable (*see* Figure 7-10, above). Barriers range from lack of engagement in the process due to comfort with the status quo to not understanding the process (process illiteracy).

*Naming the barriers.* Barriers to change usually do not simply melt away, so how can we deal with them? We can start by naming a barrier (for example, resistance, apathy) while refraining from naming an individual person. Reactions to changes range from open commitment to

public resistance.[1] We can consider these reactions as stages of readiness for change and can categorize them as follows:

- **Resistance:** Those who openly respond with behaviors and emotions to impede the change display resistance. Resistance is often the "voice" of loss or of the "threat" of loss. Exploring what is perceived as loss or a threat can be very revealing and can aid in system redesign.
- **Apathy:** Apathetic individuals show little interest in a change effort.
- **Compliance:** Those who publicly follow the changes but privately disagree with the change are compliant.
- **Commitment:** Those who are fully dedicated to the change demonstrate commitment.

Depending on the change, any one individual may be in any one of these stages. Correctly identifying the stage of readiness for change of key individuals or groups will allow the change team to understand and address the barriers that arise.

*Overcoming barriers.* Anticipating barriers to change is the key to building commitment to a change among individual staff members (*see* Table 7-3, page 127).[1] Sharing information on why a change is being made and the local historical context for the change decreases anxiety among stakeholders. It is important to anticipate how a change will affect people. The early pilot testing cycles of a change should help identify barriers. In general, people proposing change can prevent barriers by publicizing the change, providing clarity about the aim, creating excitement about the new opportunities, and showing appreciation for everyone's efforts. Note that disparaging those who resist change or those who are apathetic to change is never effective for overcoming barriers. Embracing those who resist or disagree, and working to address their concerns, demonstrates respect and develops trust while encouraging others to speak up. This approach helps those involved to develop knowledge about the system and may uncover other chances for improvement.

*What has happened/is happening with Robert, Nancy, and Bri'elle and the improvement opportunity of patients not understanding their hypertension medications? They bring a pharmacist as well as one of their clinic patients, Angela Dowling, onto their project. As you recall, they are adding the teach-back method to the clinic visit to improve patient understanding of their medications. They determine that the best team member to integrate this change concept into her daily work is the RN.*

- **Plan:** The team starts in the "Plan" phase, in which the specific goal of that test of change is stated. This is different from the overall aim of the improvement project (as discussed in Chapter 3) because the plans are very focused and directed at the immediate test of change. The Plan phase also encourages the team to create a hypothesis about what will happen when it tries this change. Finally, the Plan phase specifies who will do what, and where and when this will occur.
  - Overall global aim of the project: Improve the patients' understanding of their hypertension medications at the time of discharge.
  - Specific aim for this PDSA cycle: Increase the percentage of visits that include the use of the teach-back method for hypertension medications from 0% to 50% within the next three months.

- **Do:** Carrying out the test and documenting observations about the test occurs in the "Do" phase. The evaluation may be quantitative, qualitative, or both.
  - An additional field is added to the nursing note template to document that staff performed the teach-back method. This includes a place to document whether the patient is accurate in describing the purpose and frequency of his or her hypertension medications and a place to provide further explanation. Adding this field will facilitate the measurement of the process change to monitor improvement.

- **Study:** The "Study" phase is when the team analyzes the data. Team members summarize the results and compare them to the predicted outcome.
  - Data indicated that the teach-back method was integrated into 55% of the clinic visits for patients with hypertension. In addition, it was found that 70% of the patients had an accurate understanding of the purpose and frequency of their hypertension medications; 30% needed additional education and follow-up.

- **Act:** The "Act" phase consists of determining the consequences of the change and agreeing on the objective for the next PDSA cycle. The Act phase from one PDSA cycle flows into the Plan phase of the next cycle.
  - The team decided to keep its teach-back method in place. The team identifies that other interventions can be tested. One example is a way to manage medications at home, such as the use of a pillbox. The pillbox will help the patients identify the days and times they missed taking their medications.

## Summary

Managing change requires planning, practice, and patience. A system will not adopt a change simply because you are the clinical leader or there is a new policy; rather, successful change in complex systems is often the cumulative effect of many small changes over time. Research studies that use elegant statistical analyses often identify the individual factors that have the most influence on outcomes. Applying this information to a local setting will succeed only if the planning team understands the local culture and context. No research, no matter how closely it resembles the local setting, will be seamlessly translated to your setting. The complex adaptive nature of a system does not allow this simple implementation. Those who profess a simple translation are often assuming a simple linear relationship

| TABLE 7-3 | Strategies to Address Potential Barriers and Build Commitment for Change Within a System |
|---|---|

| Strategy | Description and Examples |
|---|---|
| 1. Provide information about the change. | • Acknowledge the anxiety that comes with change.<br>• Share the aim statement of the improvement team.<br>• Show the quality gap (via measures) that exists.<br>• Keep the patient at the center of the change efforts.<br>• Connect the change(s) to the mission and values of the organization. |
| 2. Anticipate how the change will affect people and provide this information to them. | • Be available to answer questions and accept comments.<br>• Always be prepared to study rational objections; someone may have insight that was overlooked by the team.<br>• Share results from tests of change. |
| 3. Gather information from the end users about the resources that will be necessary to make the change. | • Opinion leaders and change agents or champions are helpful, but those who are often in the late majority group or the laggard group also can provide important feedback (see Figure 7-3).<br>• Request formal and visible support from organizational leaders (for example, clinical leaders, nurse unit managers, senior administrators).<br>• Be confident about the process of testing and implementing changes and the desire to make this work with the current system. |
| 4. Publicize the change. | • Tell stories and anecdotes about successful change.<br>• Create a data board in a public space where everyone can follow the progress of the key measures.<br>• Summarize key points and agreements as they are made.<br>• Provide vocal public appreciation for those who are supportive of the change(s). |

**Source:** Adapted from Langley GJ, et al. *The Improvement Guide: A Practical Approach to Enhancing Organizational Performance*, 2nd ed. San Francisco: Jossey-Bass, 2009.

between intervention and outcome, but such simple relationships rarely occur.

This chapter focused on the last step of the Model for Improvement, following the question "What change can we make that will result in improvement?" This last step involves the use of PDSA cycles to test potential changes that will result in improvement. Potential changes may target the processes of care or may include strategies to enhance adoption, implementation, or sustainability of the change. Rogers's diffusion of innovations was presented as a useful model to provide insight into the change process. The chapter also highlighted the importance of the

identification of barriers to change so that interventions can be implemented to overcome these barriers.

Managing change is a systematic process that entails the use of evidence-based approaches as well as artful responses to local conditions. Testing and assessing a system enables a team to build knowledge about it in a rigorous and systematic way that helps generate a more reliable system. Change is not easy, but done well, it is immensely satisfying when the team is able to improve processes and outcomes in partnership with patients, families, and communities.

# References

1. Langley GJ, et al. *The Improvement Guide: A Practical Approach to Enhancing Organizational Performance*, 2nd ed. San Francisco: Jossey-Bass, 2009.

2. Institute for Healthcare Improvement. Resources. Accessed Nov 24, 2017. http://www.ihi.org/knowledge.

3. Batalden PB, Davidoff F. What is "quality improvement" and how can it transform health care? *Qual Saf Health Care*. 2007 Feb;16(1):2–3.

4. Institute of Medicine. *Crossing the Quality Chasm: A New Health System for the 21st Century*. Washington, DC: National Academy Press, 2001.

5. Plsek P. Appendix B: Redesigning health care with insights from the science of complex adaptive systems. In Institute of Medicine: *Crossing the Quality Chasm: A New Health System for the 21st Century*. Washington, DC: National Academy Press, 2001, 309–322.

6. Agency for Healthcare Research and Quality. Health Literacy Universal Precautions Toolkit, 2nd Edition: Use the Teach-Back Method: Tool #5. Feb 2015. Accessed Nov 25, 2017. https://www.ahrq.gov/professionals/quality-patient-safety/quality-resources/tools/literacy-toolkit/healthlittoolkit2-tool5.html.

7. Swift CG. Care of older people: Falls in late life and their consequences—Implementing effective services. *BMJ*. 2001 Apr 7;322(7290):855–857.

8. Rogers EM. *Diffusion of Innovations*, 4th ed. New York: Free Press, 1995.

9. Nelson EC, Batalden PB, Lazar JS, editors. *Practice-Based Learning and Improvement: A Clinical Improvement Action Guide*, 2nd ed. Oak Brook, IL: Joint Commission Resources, 2007.

10. Powell BJ, et al. A refined compilation of implementation strategies: Results from the Expert Recommendations for Implementing Change (ERIC) project. *Implement Sci*. 2015 Feb 12;10:21.

11. Proctor EK, Powell BJ, McMillen JC. Implementation strategies: Recommendations for specifying and reporting. *Implement Sci*. 2013 Dec 1;8:139.

12. Waltz TJ, et al. Use of concept mapping to characterize relationships among implementation strategies and assess their feasibility and importance: Results from the Expert Recommendations for Implementing Change (ERIC) study. *Implement Sci*. 2015 Aug 7;10:109.

13. Tomolo AM, Lawrence RH, Aron DC. A case study of translating the ACGME practice-based learning and improvement requirements into reality: Systems quality improvement projects as the key component to a comprehensive curriculum. *Postgrad Med J*. 2009 Oct;85(1008):530–537.

# Spreading Improvements

## ✓ Objectives

**After reading this chapter, you will be able to do the following:**

1. **Identify effective strategies for sustaining and spreading change.**

2. **Follow a step-by-step approach to planning spread efforts.**

3. **Avoid common mistakes and plan for success.**

## 💡 Improvement Opportunity

### The Teach-Back Method

An improvement team in a teaching hospital is very excited about improvements it has made in using teach-back with patients throughout the hospital stay to assess patients' and family caregivers' understanding of discharge instructions and ability to perform self-care. Teach-back is a method of interacting with patients to confirm that the health care provider has explained what the patient needs to know in a way that the patient understands. A patient's understanding is confirmed when he or she explains what's been said back to the health care provider.[1] It is one of the methods used to reduce the likelihood of patients returning to the hospital unnecessarily after discharge because they did not fully understand how to take care of themselves after they returned home (or because their family caregivers did not know how to administer care).[2]

The improvement team, led by nurse educator Faiza Okoye, also includes a staff nurse, a hospitalist (that is, a hospital-based physician), a pharmacist, a resident, a nursing assistant from a selected medical/surgical unit, and two patients. This inpatient team is also part of a larger cross-continuum team that's been working to reduce unnecessary readmissions to the hospital. The cross-continuum team comprises representatives from the hospital's community partners, including a local nursing home, a home health agency, a patient advocacy group, and a large primary care practice affiliated with the hospital. When interviewing patients, the inpatient improvement team quickly learned that one of the issues contributing to readmissions was that patients were often confused about which medications to take, or how to take them, when they returned home.

Faiza suggested that the team use the teach-back method to ensure that providers were appropriately explaining discharge instructions. They began by watching a teach-back video[3] and trying the method with one or two patients. Under the guidance of the nurse educator and a patient, they observed each other and learned how to interact with the patients in a more effective way. They studied how often patients could explain back what the provider had reviewed with them and improved their teach-back skills. Faiza then worked with all the nurses, residents, and nursing assistants on the unit so that all staff members who interacted with patients were confident in their use of teach-back. They were so enthusiastic about the patients' response and their own experience that they wanted to spread—to share—this new method with care teams on other units.

They presented their work to the cross-continuum team. The executive sponsor of the cross-continuum team assigned the chief nursing officer and the director of the residency program to be the leaders for spreading teach-back. The spread leaders, together with Faiza, nursing managers, residents, and the improvement team, developed a plan for spreading within the hospital that included the following components:

- The leaders and the improvement team made presentations at medical staff, residency program, patient advisory board, and unit meetings.
- The nurse educator and patient advisor developed a training schedule for units that were being introduced to teach-back, first training one or two nurses and residents who could become (with the support of the nurse managers on these units and the residency director) the mentors on the new units.

- As the mentors became capable of supporting the new units, the next five units were scheduled for training by the nurse educator.
- Data on the effectiveness of the teach-back method (such as the percentage of patients who could teach back at least 75% of the information they received) were collected in each unit by team members.
- Teach-back continued to be an agenda item at medical staff, residency program, and nursing unit meetings to reinforce its importance and to share learning about its use.
- To ensure continued use of teach-back, it was incorporated into the yearly competency training for nurses and medical assistants, as well as into the residency training program.
- Nursing, pharmacy, and medical students who spent time learning on the units were also given training so they could contribute to the teach-back efforts.

The cross-continuum team received regular updates on readmission rates and on the spread of teach-back within the hospital. Members of the cross-continuum team from community partners (nursing homes, home health agencies, area offices on aging, patient advocacy groups, and so on) saw the potential for using teach-back in their facilities and programs. With coaching from the spread leaders and Faiza, the nurse educator, they developed a plan for bringing teach-back to their staff so that patient education could be reinforced and strengthened before the patients were discharged.

# Spread: Overview and Definition

*Spread* is defined as the process by which new ideas are communicated over time through a social system,[4] with the intended outcome being the adoption of the new ideas. Spread is part of an overall process of improvement—a process that involves first testing and refining new ideas or processes on a small scale, such as in a single medical/surgical unit in a hospital or one primary care clinic, and then ensuring that the new processes are embedded in the

daily work of the clinicians and staff in those initial units (that is, ensuring that they are implemented). After the improvements have been implemented in the initial units, they are ready for broader adoption across the organization and/or to other organizations. The preceding vignette describes the adoption of the teach-back method developed in one unit by others within the hospital.

Spread sometimes occurs without much intervention, but this natural diffusion of innovation may take a long time to complete, as in the now-famous description by Everett Rogers of the spread of a new type of seed corn—in which

## DEFINED:

### Spread

*Spread* is the process by which new ideas are communicated over time through a social system, with the intended outcome being the adoption of the new ideas.

the benefits alone were not enough to promote rapid spread of its use.[4] Those involved in making care safer and better for patients want to accelerate change so it occurs as quickly as possible, because a delay in the adoption of better ideas and processes means the delivery of less-than-optimal care or the potential for patient harm. In this chapter, the term *spread* refers to a planned approach that includes the methods leaders can use to strategically plan and execute a

system that accelerates the adoption of new ideas or processes as the scope—or scale—of the change expands, and to ensure that the new ideas are sustained over time.[5]

The example we will use to illustrate a successful approach to spread is a hand hygiene initiative carried out at Iowa Health Des Moines (IHDM) to decrease infections and improve patient safety in 2008–2009.[6] The hand hygiene initiative initially involved the three hospitals that are part of IHDM: Iowa Methodist Medical Center, Blank Children's Hospital, and Iowa Lutheran Hospital. The case study in this chapter describes the initial spread processes at IHDM, which was able to achieve and sustain a 90% rate of adoption of prescribed hand hygiene policies, as compared with a 60% rate at the start of the initiative 10 months prior (*see* Figure 8-1, below).[7]

The steps in the approach included:
    Step 1: Setting a Foundation for Spread
    Step 2: Developing an Initial Plan for Spread
    Step 3: Carrying Out and Refining the Spread Plan

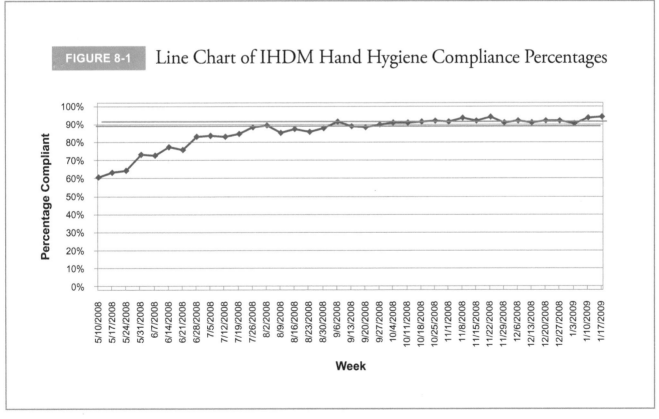

**FIGURE 8-1** Line Chart of IHDM Hand Hygiene Compliance Percentages

The above figure shows the Iowa Health Des Moines (IHDM) compliance percentages from May 2008 through January 2009, demonstrating improvement from a 60% compliance rate prior to 90% sustained after the spread processes.

**Source:** Adapted from Iowa Health Des Moines data. Printed with permission.

# Step 1: Setting a Foundation for Spread

One of the biggest mistakes that leaders make with spread initiatives is to not plan early enough for how they will spread an improvement that is developed in a pilot site. Spread does not happen without planning and preparation. There are several recommended steps to consider in establishing a solid foundation for spread,[5] including establishing a team to lead the spread effort and ensuring alignment between the strategic goals of the organization and the spread effort. It is important to note here that the primary responsibility for planning and organizing spread rests with the leadership of the organization or system. Frontline staff play an important role in spread; they are members of teams where the improvements are tested and refined so they can be easily shared with others. The support structure needed to spread changes across a system must be established, supported, and maintained by the leadership.

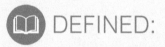 DEFINED:

**Spread Team**
A *spread team* is a group established by an organization's leaders to guide and monitor a spread effort.

## Establishing a Spread Team

A *spread team* is a group established by an organization's leaders to guide and monitor a spread effort. The senior leaders at IHDM established an interprofessional team to identify and carry out improvements in the system's hand hygiene processes. The team included the following members:

- **Team sponsors:** The executive director of women's services and the director of clinical quality provided resources, support, and encouragement to the IHDM team.

- **Day-to-day leader:** The person responsible for the day-to-day activities of the team was an infection prevention nurse at IHDM. This person—who

functioned as the spread team leader—convened team meetings, helped the team make and carry out its plans, kept track of tests that were under way, ensured that the data needed to support the team's work were collected and displayed, and provided update reports to senior leaders.

- **Facilitator:** The quality improvement coordinator, acting as facilitator, helped to ensure that team meetings were well organized and productive and that all members of the team contributed to its work and progress. The coordinator also assisted the leader in keeping track of tests, data, and reports.

- **Team leaders:** Two physician leaders (the hospital epidemiologist and the vice president of medical affairs) promoted the initiative among physicians during medical staff meetings and followed up personally with other physician leaders and individual physicians, as needed, throughout the initiative.

- **Other clinicians and staff:** Members included clinicians and staff members who were involved in initially identifying, testing, and refining changes to improve hand washing in the initial units, as well as representatives from the target units in each hospital. They included nurse supervisors and managers from medical and surgical services, oncology, rehabilitation, critical care, behavioral health, and the emergency department; a resident; and representatives from marketing, epidemiology, and environmental services.

## Aligning a Spread Effort with Strategic Goals

For spread to be successful, leadership needs to provide a clear and unambiguous message that the status quo is unacceptable and that the improvements to be spread are central to the success of the organization. When the chief medical officer established a corporate clinical performance improvement department responsible for quality performance and clinical safety improvement across the system, IHDM dedicated itself to improving patient safety.[7]

Before IHDM began the hand hygiene initiative, The Joint Commission noted lapses in hand hygiene during a resurvey. This got the attention of the system's leaders. The chief executive officer, other members of the executive team, and managers across IHDM sent a clear message through written and verbal communication channels that hand hygiene was a priority for the organization and that process changes should be developed by interprofessional teams and spread across IHDM. To emphasize the importance of this effort, hospital leaders visited units and departments to listen to and encourage staff as the changes in the hand hygiene process were initiated and spread by the organization.

## Establishing a Spread Aim

A *spread aim* is a clear, concise statement of what an organization intends to accomplish. A good spread aim should address what is being spread, the target audience or population, the time frame, and the expected level of improvement—essentially, the "what," "who," "when," and "how much" of spread. In April 2008 the spread team at IHDM developed an aim statement: "Iowa Health–Des Moines employees will demonstrate 90% compliance with hand hygiene opportunities by August 1, 2008. Executive directors and managers will be sent weekly reports on hand hygiene compliance in their areas and will follow up with employees. They will send a clear message that hand hygiene is a top priority for patient care at IHDM."

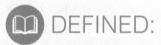 DEFINED:

### Spread Aim
A *spread aim* is a clear, concise statement of what an organization intends to accomplish.

The expectations for hand hygiene were clearly spelled out in a hand hygiene policy that had originally been developed by the organization several years earlier and then revised prior to the launch of the hand hygiene spread effort. The policy was used as the basis for determining compliance for the spread aim.

# Step 2: Developing an Initial Plan for Spread

The spread plan addresses the question of how the organization will reach the goals outlined in the spread aim. There are a number of methods that can be used to organize spread activities, including everything from large-scale campaigns to the use of extension agents working locally.[8] The appropriate method depends on the level of resources (time and money), the characteristics of the organizational structure (such as centralized or decentralized), and the expected reception of the new ideas (resistance, skepticism, and so on).

*Spread plan elements.* The methods for spread may differ, but there are elements that are common among them that must be included in any successful spread effort:

- A communication system to share information and resources
- A way to connect the people to maximize learning and support
- A measurement system to track progress and results
- A process for making adjustments in the spread plan, as needed

Leaders at IHDM used an already established process for chartering teams (for example, the hand hygiene team) to develop solutions to quality and safety problems and then spread them across their system, using the facility, department, and unit structure to imbed the new practices. They called the effort the One Touch Campaign, as a way to generate interest and energy and to emphasize its importance.

The spread team at IHDM went out and asked those at the bedside and in the ancillary areas at each hospital what beliefs they had about hand hygiene and what they perceived as barriers to cleaning their hands. They found two important factors that were contributing to less-than-optimal hand washing:

- The gel containers weren't refilled promptly and/or they weren't used because the gel created skin problems for staff.
- Many staff and clinicians believed that using gloves took the place of cleaning hands, not understanding that putting gloves on with unwashed hands would leave germs on the outside of the gloves and pose a risk to patients.

To address these issues, the spread team worked with the distributor to replace gel with foam and installed 1,800 new foam container holders (which IHDM received for free from the manufacturer), including one in and one outside every room to ensure that they were conveniently located. Even though mounting that many new container holders in more convenient locations was challenging, staff were able to complete the work in three weeks, reflecting the priority of the campaign for the hospitals. The spread team also addressed the misperception about using gloves through an educational program that was part of the team's larger communication plan (described in the following section).

## Developing a Communication Plan

A good communication plan is needed for any spread effort to fulfill its two primary purposes: (1) build awareness of the new ideas and (2) provide technical knowledge and support to those ready to adopt the ideas. The purposes should be matched with the appropriate methods of communication.[9] For example, large meetings may help to build awareness, while one-to-one conversations may be more effective for moving people closer to the decision to adopt or to provide details about how to make the improvements.

> **66 99** **Large meetings may help to build awareness, while one-to-one conversations may be more effective for moving people closer to the decision to adopt or to provide details about how to make the improvements.**

The communication plan that the spread team used did the following:

- It built awareness by holding a systemwide kickoff event and developing and displaying 1,000 posters in prominent locations throughout the hospitals (including on each unit).
- It provided technical knowledge about correct hand-washing techniques and principles through online educational modules (which included signing a hand hygiene pledge) that all staff were required to complete.
- It incorporated a hand hygiene policy into the curriculum for the spread effort. In addition, the infection prevention and control nurse leader and hospital epidemiologist worked directly with the residents on infection prevention and control, emphasizing hand hygiene. The educational curriculum also addressed two other important aspects of communication: making the case for why a change is important and simplifying the steps needed to adopt the change. The training emphasized the importance of correct hand hygiene techniques, including why it is important to clean one's hands before putting on gloves and how the foam containers were changed to make it easier for staff to follow the hand hygiene policy.

### Addressing response to change

Smart communication strategies address how potential adopters will view the new way of doing things. Rogers identified five characteristics of an innovation that can contribute to the rate of adoption of a new idea or process: the perceived relative advantage of the change; the complexity of the change; its compatibility with the culture, values, and structures currently in place; how observable the new process is to potential adopters; and whether adopters can try the process before committing to its implementation.[4] Through its communication methods and messages, the spread team presented the hand hygiene techniques as practices that would result in fewer infections for patients, as something relatively simple and easy to do (for example, the foam container holders were placed conveniently in and near patient rooms), and as easily observable to both staff and patients. After the policy was established, the spread team continued to gather information as staff took steps to follow the policy and incorporate its practices into daily work flows (that is, making the change "trialable").

## Using the Social System for Spread

The social system for spread includes the individuals and groups in the target population—that is, the staff in the locations where the transition from the old system to the new one takes place. Spread is successful when a new idea or process is adopted by the members of the social system in the target population. However, because individuals in a social system do not necessarily adopt changes at the same time (as Rogers identified and as described in Chapter 7), moving new ideas from a successful site to the target population is not always a simple process.

The spread team at IHDM had two strategies to maximize relationships in the social system to accelerate spread: (1) using the department and unit structure and (2) removing environmental barriers.

### Using the department and unit structure

The IHDM spread team used the organization's department and unit structure to reach all staff and clinicians, including nurses, physicians, residents, environmental services, ancillary services, and the emergency department. Each nurse manager took charge of his or her unit's performance, ensuring that nurses and all staff members were aware of and followed the hand-washing policies. In addition, physician leaders played an important role in communicating with other physicians. For example, when the spread team made the head of a major ancillary department aware of the data in his department, he immediately reinforced the new processes with his physicians. Also, the resident on the spread team served as a liaison among the spread team, the residents, and the physicians. All staff were encouraged not only to clean their own hands but also to give feedback to any physicians, nurses, or residents who were not following the hand-hygiene process. Clinical faculty also communicated and reinforced the hand-washing policies with the residents.

## Removing environmental barriers

As discussed earlier, the spread team at IHDM identified an environmental and structural issue: the installation of new foam containers. Such structural issues, or transition issues, can slow individuals' willingness to adopt new ideas.[10] Installing functional containers at appropriate sites removed some barriers. Other examples of such obstacles include features of the information system, staffing policies or procedures, and compensation or reimbursement systems. It is the responsibility of the spread leaders to "listen" to the target population to understand barriers to adoption and develop ways to overcome them.[11]

# Measurement

A measurement system for spread includes the main outcome measures of the process or system of interest and the rate of spread of the specific improvements. In addition to the measurement system, a feedback system is needed to provide information on progress in reaching the organization's spread goals to the executive leadership, the spread team, and the adopters in the target population.

## Collecting the data

The spread team at IHDM developed a hand hygiene–monitoring tool and then took it to various areas of the hospitals to get feedback. The team revised the tool based on that feedback and selected monitors on each of the units. In each of the three hospitals, a manager on each unit and ancillary unit chose someone to do the monitoring—someone who really believed in what hand hygiene can do for infection rates. Each monitor received education on how to complete the observations and collect the data. To reduce the burden of data collection and reporting, the monitors counted 10 "before–patient contact" and 10 "after–patient contact" opportunities each week and entered their data using an online survey tool. The monitors sent data results to all units in the form of weekly reports. Also included in the weekly report were job codes across the board—from physicians to nursing and all ancillary staff—so that reports showed the performance of all staff by job category.

## Sharing the data

Each unit prominently displayed the data, and staff discussed the data's implications. If the data indicated a lack of compliance with the hand–hygiene policy, the unit manager, department director, or physician leader would follow up with members of the unit or department.

## Accountability for the data

Units were held accountable by anyone who visited their unit—not just their own staff. So if someone, staff or visitor, was on a unit, he or she counted in the observations for that unit. This created an environment of accountability in the units so that unit staff felt responsible for what went on in their own units.

## Responding to the data

Sharing data openly sent the message that the data would be used by the hospital for improvement rather than for judgment. The spread team purposely asked leadership not to impose punitive measures on staff who didn't clean their hands. Leaders approached the campaign as a collaborative effort with staff, viewing it as an opportunity for employee growth and enhanced competence.

 **Sharing data openly sent the message that the data would be used by the hospital for improvement rather than for judgment.**

Because the focus of the campaign was on hand hygiene, the measure of interest (in this case, the outcome measure) that the organization tracked was compliance with the hand-hygiene policy for all three hospitals combined—with a goal of 90%. The process measure was the completion of 10 "before–" and "after–" patient contact opportunities by the monitors, with a goal of 100% of the monitoring counts being completed. An additional measure the spread team observed to ensure that staff were not suffering adverse skin effects from the hand washing and cleansing was the skin conditions of staff hands, as reported on two staff surveys over a period of a year.

Positive reinforcement was an important part of the campaign as well. The units that met the goal of 90% were highlighted in the weekly e-mails, and their data were attached. Unit celebrations and other events were held by unit managers to recognize achievement and to build energy and enthusiasm. For example, to add some fun to the campaign, two nurse managers dressed as clowns and visited top-performing units with a wagon full of candy. System leaders also got involved in the celebration. The chief operations officer and another administrator made the rounds in a "hand" costume, complimenting people cleaning their hands as they went.

After a period of eight months, the spread team and hospital leaders started highlighting the units that were not meeting hand-hygiene compliance in the weekly e-mail. To sustain the improvements (and to ensure that the hand-hygiene policy was embedded in unit and department processes and culture), the spread team continued to do weekly measurement of hand hygiene for a year. Then, for four months, the team switched to collecting the data every two weeks. Following that, the team collected data monthly for six months. Eventually the team began collecting and publishing data every quarter.

# Step 3: Carrying Out and Refining the Spread Plan

It is the responsibility of the spread team to gather information about the spread process as it unfolds in the organization. The spread team plays an important role in monitoring the process and recommending adjustments, as needed, to ensure the meeting of spread goals. Communication plans, materials and information, support and mentorship, infrastructure issues, and social system issues all may need attention during a spread effort.

To gather information about how the campaign was progressing, the leaders of the IHDM spread team visited the units, identifying issues with the monitoring process and barriers that surfaced. For example, the spread leaders followed up with unit managers and physician leaders when the data indicated a lack of awareness or other issues contributing to low monitoring scores.

## Sustaining Improvement

Part of the work of refining and strengthening the spread plan involves taking action to ensure that the changes made during a spread effort are sustained over time. IHDM built a number of actions into its campaign that contributed to the high level of hand hygiene the organization was able to sustain over time, including the following:

- It established and documented standard processes in the hand-hygiene policy.
- It set the expectation that hand hygiene is a standard part of every staff member's and clinician's daily responsibilities.
- It used ongoing monitoring, data collection, and reporting to keep the focus on following the policy.

- It developed an online educational module to ensure that all current and new staff would have a solid foundation in the hand-hygiene policy.
- It assigned ownership initially through the spread team; after a year and a half, the organization transferred responsibility for monitoring and follow-up to operational and managerial leaders.
- It addressed the social aspects of change by using positive reinforcement, incorporated a fun culture into the campaign, and celebrated and recognized high-performing units and departments.

## Recommended Spread Effort Components

The following are recommended components for leaders to consider in planning and carrying out successful spread efforts:

- Agenda setting and active involvement of leaders, including a designated spread team
- A clear aim, with measurable targets and a time line
- A spread plan that includes a set of ideas or practices, a way to attract and support adopters, thoughtful use of the social system and attention to structural issues, a measurement and feedback system, and a method to refine the plan, as needed
- Hardwiring of new practices into established policies and procedures, monitoring and tracking of results over time, and attention to cultural issues so that staff, providers, and trainees continue to learn, grow, and feel connected to the ongoing improvements over time

The Institute for Healthcare Improvement (IHI) white paper, *A Framework for Spread*,[8] provides more detail about these components and serves as a guide for leaders to use in incorporating the following into their spread strategy: the role of leadership, the organizational setup to support spread, the description of the new ideas, methods of communication, nurturing of the social system, measurement and feedback systems, and knowledge management. The framework (*see* Figure 8-2 on page 137) is not prescriptive. Rather, it suggests some general areas for an organization or a team to consider as it undertakes a spread project. Through effective spread, organizations share and adopt improvements more broadly, contributing to improved performance by the organization or system and ultimately to health care improvement.

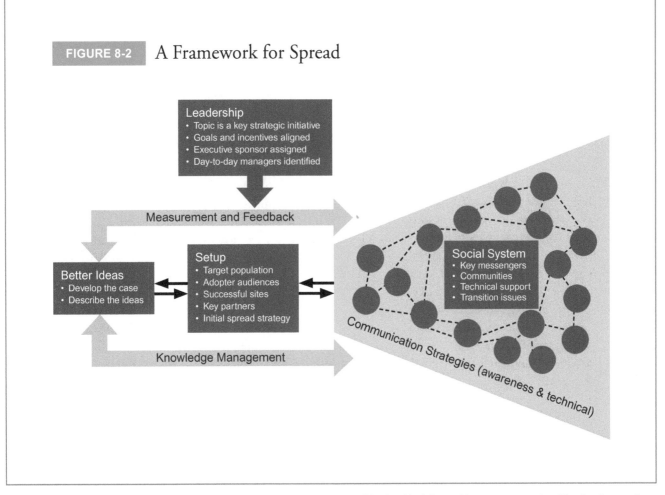

FIGURE 8-2 A Framework for Spread

**Leadership**
• Topic is a key strategic initiative
• Goals and incentives aligned
• Executive sponsor assigned
• Day-to-day managers identified

Measurement and Feedback

**Better Ideas**
• Develop the case
• Describe the ideas

**Setup**
• Target population
• Adopter audiences
• Successful sites
• Key partners
• Initial spread strategy

**Social System**
• Key messengers
• Communities
• Technical support
• Transition issues

Communication Strategies (awareness & technical)

Knowledge Management

This diagram illustrates the intersection of ideas with setup, social system, and leadership, informed by measurement and feedback as well as knowledge management.

Source: Nolan K, et al. Using a framework for spread: The case of patient access in the Veterans Health Administration. *Jt Comm J Qual Patient Saf.* 2005 Jun;31(6):339–347. Used with permission.

# Summary

The experience of IHDM in launching and supporting a successful spread effort to improve hand hygiene illustrates a number of key features that can help an organization achieve its goals and sustain improvement over time. Planning and leading spread efforts is the responsibility of an organization's leaders, but staff, clinicians, and even trainees play important roles in testing, refining, and helping others to understand and adopt new ideas and processes.

## Spread Through Learner and Patient/ Family Networks

Learners can contribute substantially to the spread of clinical improvement through grassroots efforts like those of the IHI Open School to spread the use of the World Health

Organization (WHO) Surgical Safety Checklist.[12] Learners can also contribute to spread of population-based improvement through change agency structures like the IHI Open School Change Agent Network (I-CAN).[13] Recognizing that universities were not equipping health professional students to address the social determinants of health, I-CAN sought to engage 30,000 individuals in actions to improve population health in their local settings when it launched in 2014.

These actions would require students to move beyond the walls of their clinics, to address the root causes of problems in patients' lives. One mechanism for developing this "army of change agents" is an innovative, project-based I-CAN online course, "Leadership and Organizing for Change."[14] The course teaches skills in leadership and community organizing as well as expertise in the drivers of population health. Course participants leverage approaches such as storytelling, strategic relationship-building, distributing leadership, and interprofessional teamwork to engage their classmates and community members in collective actions related to population health—whether that involves a pledge to avoid texting and driving, getting a flu shot on campus, or engaging new caregivers in best practices in newborn care. By the end of the initial 16-month campaign, IHI Open School student leaders had catalyzed more than 35,000 individuals to take action to improve population health. Since the fall of 2014, more than 1,600 learners have engaged with the Leadership and Organizing for Change course, which continues to build capacity for student leadership in the Open School and beyond.[14,15]

Spread efforts may also extend beyond health care institutions. For example, ImproveCareNow[16] is a network of providers, researchers, patients, and parents who engage in improvement efforts for the treatment of pediatric inflammatory bowel disease across the nation. Developed as a model for improving subspecialty care through the sponsorship of the North American Society for Pediatric Gastroenterology, Hepatology and Nutrition and the American Board of Pediatrics, the effort includes three components: (1) creating multicenter collaborative networks of pediatric subspecialists, (2) sharing performance data from patient registries, and (3) training in quality improvement. The network first focused on improving diagnosis, classifying disease severity, detecting and treating inadequate nutrition and growth, and dosing of medications. Ten practice sites started in 2007, and the network grew to 24 sites by 2010. More than 2,500 patients were enrolled in the registry by 2009, resulting in data from more than 7,500 visits. Sites are making improvements not only in care processes, but also in important outcomes such as remission rates.[17] ImproveCareNow's infrastructure for spread includes an online portal, a registry, and a knowledge exchange commons. Parents also use social media outlets to extend beyond the professional exchange and reach parents and caregivers outside the network.

Spreading change is challenging, but success is possible by setting the foundation, developing a plan, carrying out and refining the plan, and engaging a broad range of stakeholders, including learners and patients, families, and communities.

# References

1. Agency for Healthcare Research and Quality. Health Literacy Universal Precautions Toolkit, 2nd ed. Berga AG, et al. Feb 2015. Accessed Nov 25, 2017. https://www.ahrq.gov/professionals/quality-patient-safety/quality-resources/tools/literacy-toolkit/healthlittoolkit2.html.

2. Schillinger D, et al. Closing the loop: Physician communication with diabetic patients who have low health literacy. *Arch Intern Med.* 2003 Jan 13:163(1):83–90.

3. Institute for Healthcare Improvement Open School. *What Is Teach-Back?* 2016. Video. Accessed Dec 11, 2017. https://www.youtube.com/watch?v=bzpJJYF_tKY.

4. Rogers EM. *Diffusion of Innovations*, 4th ed. New York: Free Press, 1995.

5. Nolan KM, Schall MW. A framework for spread. In Nolan KM, Schall MW, editors: *Spreading Improvement Across Your Health Care Organization*. Oak Brook, IL: Joint Commission Resources; Cambridge, MA: Institute for Healthcare Improvement, 2007, 1–24.

6. Personal communication between the author and Pat Busick, MS, CIA, Iowa Lutheran Hospital, and Julie Gibbons, RN, BSN, CIC, Iowa Health Des Moines, Feb 18, 2011.

7. Nolan K, Nielsen GA, Schall MW. Developing strategies to spread improvements. In Joint Commission on Accreditation of Healthcare Organizations: *From Front Office to Front Line: Essential Issues for Health Care Leaders*. Oakbrook Terrace, IL: Joint Commission Resources, 2005, 145–176.

8. Massoud MR, et al. *A Framework for Spread: From Local Improvements to System-Wide Change.* IHI Innovation Series white paper. Cambridge, MA: Institute for Healthcare Improvement, 2006. Accessed Nov 25, 2017. http://www.ihi.org/resources/Pages/IHIWhitePapers/AFrameworkforSpreadWhitePaper.aspx.

9. Fraser SW. *Accelerating the Spread of Good Practice: A Workbook for Health Care.* Chicester, UK: Kingsham Press, 2002.

10. Brown JS, Duguid P. *The Social Life of Information.* Boston: Harvard Business School Press, 2000.

11. Dixon NM. Common Knowledge: *How Companies Thrive by Sharing What They Know.* Boston: Harvard Business School Press, 2000.

12. Henderson D, et al. Check a box. Save a life: How student leadership is shaking up health care and driving a revolution in patient safety. *J Patient Saf.* 2010 Mar;6(1):43–47.

13. Institute for Healthcare Improvement. IHI Open School: IHI Open School Change Agent Network (I-CAN). Accessed Nov 25, 2017. http://www.ihi.org/education/IHIOpenSchool/ICAN/Pages/default.aspx.

14. Institute for Healthcare Improvement. Virtual Training: Leadership and Organizing for Change. Accessed Nov 25, 2017. http://www.ihi.org/education/WebTraining/Webinars/LeadershipOrganizing/Pages/default.aspx.

15. Institute for Healthcare Improvement. Made to Stick: Open School Presentation. Oct 2017. Accessed Nov 25, 2017. http://www.ihi.org/education/IHIOpenSchool/Chapters/Documents/Made%20To%20Stick%20IHI%20Open%20School%20Presentation_Oct2017.pptx.

16. ImproveCareNow. Home page. Accessed Nov 25, 2017. http://www.improvecarenow.org/.

17. Crandall W, et al. ImproveCareNow: The development of a pediatric inflammatory bowel disease improvement network. *Inflamm Bowel Dis*. 2011 Jan;17(1):450–457.

# Publishing, Presenting, and Teaching Quality Improvement

## ✔ Objectives

**After reading this chapter, you will be able to do the following:**

1. **Describe how to use the SQUIRE 2.0 guidelines to be more successful in publishing your improvement work.**

2. **Identify educational principles essential to developing learning experiences in improvement.**

3. **Appreciate developmental levels in implementing improvement curricula for health care professionals.**

4. **Describe examples of learning experiences in improvement.**

"What I hear, I forget.
What I see, I remember.
What I do, I understand."

—Confucius

## 💡 Improvement Opportunity

### Dissemination Opportunity

Jennifer Sorensen, an attending hospitalist in the internal medicine department; Tomas Muñoz, a nurse educator working in a medical unit; and Maureen Cox, inpatient hospital patient/family representative and improvement team member, are all very excited. As coworkers in a medical unit in a major academic medical center, Jennifer and Tomas find their jobs challenging and stimulating. Their focus is on caring for patients, but they also enjoy working with medical and nursing students who are eager to learn, ask thought-provoking questions, and contribute to patient care. Now Jennifer, Tomas, and Maureen have a new opportunity to improve the quality of care and teach at the same time; they realize they can integrate the improvement of health care into the delivery and teaching of patient care.

As members of the hospital's rapid response team (RRT) for improvement, Jennifer and Tomas saw improvement in action for the first time, with a one-third reduction in the hospital cardiac arrest rate since the implementation of the RRT a year earlier. Maureen's sister was one of these patients. Maureen witnessed the system firsthand and is eager to be a partner in improving the RRT. Patients who otherwise might have died were surviving and leaving the hospital. The trio can now see how working on improvement across professions makes it possible to provide better, more-individualized care, patient by patient. For example, thanks to the RRT protocol, a patient—Mrs. Monomuro—was transferred into the intensive care unit (ICU) much faster than she would have been in the old "call the ICU fellow" days. At the same time, care has improved for an entire group of patients—people who, like Mrs. Monomuro, might otherwise have progressed to a cardiac arrest.

Many RRT interventions have been reported in the health care literature, but the RRT improvement team can find no published reports describing the inclusion of patients' family members as a core part of the team. Theirs might be the first. Maureen's direct input, perspective on data, and guidance about possible improvements made the local changes more robust and sustainable. Amit Chandra, the ICU pharmacist who leads the improvement team, is now directing a writing group to report the work in a presentation at a national meeting and in a peer-reviewed journal using the Standards for Quality Improvement Reporting Excellence (SQUIRE 2.0) publication guidelines.

# Using a Structured Framework to Design and Disseminate Improvement Work

Working on the improvement of health care services can be fulfilling. Busy frontline professionals creating local change and making care better for patients is at the heart of professional responsibilities. However, those who work in academic medical centers are often looking for something extra and may have additional expectations as part of their work duties. How can you publish your improvement work in peer-reviewed literature or present the work at a regional, national, or international meeting?

The reality is that many journals, editors, and peer reviewers are still skeptical about publishing reports of improvement efforts because it is methodologically different than traditionally published research articles in the intent, methods, and analysis. Research seeks to create new generalizable evidence, while improvement seeks to create system-level changes that implement evidence-based practices for patients. In addition, many individuals involved in improvement work do not have writing experience or incentives, so reporting their efforts is challenging.

In 2008 the SQUIRE guidelines were published[1], providing an opportunity to share improvement work in the scholarly literature. These guidelines were used widely by professionals seeking publication, and as the field of improvement developed, the guidelines were revised (SQUIRE 2.0) to improve the transparency and completeness of published reports about systematic efforts to improve the quality, safety, and value of health care services.[2]

SQUIRE 2.0 (http://www.squire-statement.org) offers guidance on reporting original studies of quality improvement (QI). It explicitly acknowledges the context dependence, complexity, and iterative nature of improvement work. SQUIRE 2.0 balances measuring the impact of the improvement work ("Did we make the system better?") with discovery and explanation of the mechanisms at work ("How do we know improved because of our intervention[s]?"). The intent of the revised guidelines is to support the planning as well as the writing phase of improvement work. Scholarly efforts to improve the quality, safety, and value of health care services must be conducted with a high level of rigor.

## SQUIRE 2.0

What is in the guidelines that is similar to or different from other publication guidelines? SQUIRE 2.0 consists of "Notes to Authors" and 19 individual items to consider when writing a complete report of improvement work (see Table 9-1). It builds on the familiar Introduction, Methods, Results, and Discussion (IMRaD) format used in most health care journals. Importantly, authors should consider every SQUIRE item, but it may be inappropriate or unnecessary to include every SQUIRE element in a particular manuscript.

SQUIRE 2.0 contains three unique elements. First, it recommends the use of a clear *rationale* (see Table 9-1, item 5). This may be a formal or informal framework, a model, or a theory to explain the assumptions used and the reasons the authors expected the intervention(s) to work. Ideally, this is determined before the work has commenced. Second, SQUIRE 2.0 encourages the assessment and reporting of the *context*. This begins in the methods section with a description of the initial contextual elements (see Table 9-1, item 7) and continues as the author(s) describes how the context affected the intervention, the

| **TABLE 9-1** | Revised Standards for Quality Improvement Reporting Excellence (SQUIRE 2.0) |
|---|---|

| **Notes to Authors** | |
|---|---|

- The SQUIRE guidelines provide a framework for reporting new knowledge about how to improve healthcare.
- The SQUIRE guidelines are intended for reports that describe system-level work to improve the quality, safety, and value of health care, and used methods to establish that observed outcomes were due to the intervention(s).
- A range of approaches exists for improving health care. SQUIRE may be adapted for reporting any of these.
- Authors should consider every SQUIRE item, but it may be inappropriate or unnecessary to include every SQUIRE element in a particular manuscript.
- The SQUIRE Glossary contains definitions of many of the key words in SQUIRE.
- The Explanation and Elaboration document provides specific examples of well-written SQUIRE items, and an in-depth explanation of each item.
- Please cite SQUIRE when it is used to write a manuscript.

| **Title and Abstract** | |
|---|---|
| **1. Title** | Indicate that the manuscript concerns an initiative to improve health care (broadly defined to include the quality, safety, effectiveness, patient-centeredness, timeliness, cost, efficiency, and equity of health care) |
| **2. Abstract** | a. Provide adequate information to aid in searching and indexing |
| | b. Summarize all key information from various sections of the text using the abstract format of the intended publication or a structured summary such as: background, local problem, methods, interventions, results, conclusions |
| **Introduction** | *Why did you start?* |
| **3. Problem Description** | Nature and significance of the local problem |
| **4. Available Knowledge** | Summary of what is currently known about the problem, including relevant previous studies |
| **5. Rationale** | Informal or formal frameworks, models, concepts, and/or theories used to explain the problem, any reasons or assumptions that were used to develop the intervention(s), and reasons why the intervention(s) was expected to work |
| **6. Specific Aims** | Purpose of the project and of this report |

| TABLE 9-1 | Revised Standards for Quality Improvement Reporting Excellence (SQUIRE 2.0) *(continued)* |
|---|---|
| **Methods** | *What did you do?* |
| 7. **Context** | Contextual elements considered important at the outset of introducing the intervention(s) |
| 8. **Intervention(s)** | a. Description of the intervention(s) in sufficient detail that others could reproduce it<br>b. Specifics of the team involved in the work |
| 9. **Study of the Intervention(s)** | a. Approach chosen for assessing the impact of the intervention(s)<br>b. Approach used to establish whether the observed outcomes were due to the intervention(s) |
| 10. **Measures** | a. Measures chosen for studying processes and outcomes of the intervention(s), including rationale for choosing them, their operational definitions, and their validity and reliability<br>b. Description of the approach to the ongoing assessment of contextual elements that contributed to the success, failure, efficiency, and cost<br>c. Methods employed for assessing completeness and accuracy of data |
| 11. **Analysis** | a. Qualitative and quantitative methods used to draw inferences from the data<br>b. Methods for understanding variation within the data, including the effects of time as a variable |
| 12. **Ethical Considerations** | Ethical aspects of implementing and studying the intervention(s) and how they were addressed, including, but not limited to, formal ethics review and potential conflict(s) of interest |
| **Results** | *What did you find?* |
| 13. **Results** | a. Initial steps of the intervention(s) and their evolution over time (e.g., time-line diagram, flowchart, or table), including modifications made to the intervention during the project<br>b. Details of the process measures and outcome<br>c. Contextual elements that interacted with the intervention(s)<br>d. Observed associations between outcomes, interventions, and relevant contextual elements<br>e. Unintended consequences such as unexpected benefits, problems, failures, or costs associated with the intervention(s)<br>f. Details about missing data |

TABLE 9-1 Revised Standards for Quality Improvement Reporting Excellence (SQUIRE 2.0) *(continued)*

| Discussion | What does it mean? |
|---|---|
| **14. Summary** | a. Key findings, including relevance to the rationale and specific aims<br>b. Particular strengths of the project |
| **15. Interpretation** | a. Nature of the association between the intervention(s) and the outcomes<br>b. Comparison of results with findings from other publications<br>c. Impact of the project on people and systems<br>d. Reasons for any differences between observed and anticipated outcomes, including the influence of context<br>e. Costs and strategic trade-offs, including opportunity costs |
| **16. Limitations** | 1. Limits to the generalizability of the work<br>2. Factors that might have limited internal validity such as confounding, bias, or imprecision in the design, methods, measurement, or analysis<br>3. Efforts made to minimize and adjust for limitations |
| **17. Conclusions** | a. Usefulness of the work<br>b. Sustainability<br>c. Potential for spread to other contexts<br>d. Implications for practice and for further study in the field<br>e. Suggested next steps |
| **Other Information** | |
| **18. Funding** | Sources of funding that supported this work. Role, if any, of the funding organization in the design, implementation, interpretation, and reporting |

**Source:** SQUIRE. Revised Standards for Quality Improvement Reporting Excellence: SQUIRE 2.0. Accessed Nov 26, 2017. http://squire-statement.org/index.cfm?fuseaction=Page.ViewPage&pageId=471. Printed with permission from BMJ Publishing Group Limited.

measurement, and ultimately the results and discussion. Third, the guidelines encourage a clear *study of the intervention(s)* (*see* Table 9-1, item 9), which describes the approach chosen for assessing the impact and establishing whether the observed outcomes were due, in fact, to the intervention(s).

## Rationale

It is important to construct a rationale at the beginning of improvement work. Researchers use theoretical frameworks, models, logic diagrams, and other tools to explain why they believe their interventions will be effective.[3] Researchers do

this whether they are working on microscopic cell cultures or designing a clinical trial of a new medication. Most improvement also contains a rationale, but it is often implicit or hidden. Improvement work can be more effective by addressing these assumptions and hunches explicitly. Examples of improvement rationale include the following:

1. Creating a reminder in the electronic health record will induce primary care physicians to order appropriate health screening tests.
2. Using posters and other print materials will enable families to initiate an RRT to evaluate their family

member; this will decrease ICU transfers and increase patient and family satisfaction of the care.

3. Creating an automatic order set for hospitalized patients will decrease the variation in ordering, increase communication among the health care team, and increase the use of evidence-based preventive measures such as regular repositioning of patients to prevent pressure ulcers.

Note that these examples reveal an anticipated causal chain of what the improvement team hypothesized will occur from the proposed intervention(s). Clarifying the rationale at the outset assists with identifying appropriate measures, modifying the intervention(s) in each Plan–Do–Study–Act (PDSA) cycle, assessing the effectiveness of the work, and planning the next set of interventions.[3] While the aim of the improvement work focuses on *what* the team wants to achieve, the rationale describes *how* the team expects the intervention(s) to work. These are complementary to each other. Authors may express a rationale in an improvement manuscript with a simple sentence (as in the examples above) or through a formal theoretical construct like a driver diagram.

## Context

This book introduced context in Chapter 4 with a discussion that highlighted the importance of understanding, studying, and sharing the contextual elements in which improvement occurs. When seeking to publish improvement work, describing the contextual elements is key for readers to understand whether the intervention(s) will be applicable to their local environments. Describing the context well leads to better replicability of the work. In the SQUIRE 2.0 guidelines, context is represented as its own item (#7) and is woven throughout several of the other items such as Measures (#10), Results (#13), Interpretation (#15), and Conclusions (#17) (*see* Table 9-1).

*Context* is defined in SQUIRE 2.0 as the physical and sociocultural makeup of the local environment and the interpretation of these factors by the health care delivery professionals, patients, and caregivers that can impact the effectiveness and generalizability of the intervention(s).[2] Context is more than just a description of the physical setting. It includes all the things that affect your intervention(s) and may include factors that are external (incentives, leadership, culture) and internal (improvement experience/skill within the microsystem, data availability, collaboration across professions). Accurately describing the context requires diligent studying of it during the improvement work. This might be done through observation, surveys, interviews, or other instruments.

Writing about the impact of context is writing about the balance between the facilitating forces and the constraining forces that either assist the intervention(s) to be effective or do not. Currently, there is no perfect "context instrument" available, but there are several frameworks in the published literature that may be helpful, such as the Promoting Action on Research Implementation in Health Services (PARIHS) framework[4] and the Consolidated Framework for Implementation Research (CFIR).[5]

## Study of the intervention

Studying the intervention(s) is often a very challenging aspect of scholarly improvement. Studying the intervention is really stepping back from the "doing" of the improvement and formally "studying" it. It answers the questions "Did the observed changes occur because of your intervention(s)? Did your intervention(s) work for the reasons you thought it did?" Studying the improvement requires a diligent and rigorous approach to understanding what happened and why it happened. If you report only the outcomes of the improvement, then readers do not know about what else might have affected the processes and outcomes. These other influences might be the Hawthorne effect (gets better because the improvement team is watching or paying attention), trends that occur within health care and society, cultural shifts, or external pressures. There are many, many influences on every system, so studying the intervention(s) teases apart the effect of the intervention(s) from other possible influences.

Studying the intervention(s) should not be conflated with requiring a research design. Certainly, improvement that employs a component of a research design such as stratified randomization or other research designs can be one way to study the effect of the intervention(s). But these more advanced designs require training and expertise. Studying the intervention(s) can be done with detailed process assessment and modeling (Chapter 4), thorough assessment of participants and nonparticipants, or even an economic evaluation to determine whether the benefit of the intervention(s) was worth the cost. There are many options to understand the impacts of the intervention(s), and doing this well is one of the unique elements of scholarly improvement that will enhance the likelihood of peer-reviewed publication.

## Other resources in the guidelines

The SQUIRE website (http://www.squire-statement.org) contains additional helpful resources. The online table of the SQUIRE 2.0 guidelines links to a glossary of terms. Many terms in the SQUIRE 2.0 guidelines are common (such as "system" or "problem"), but also have nuances that may cause misunderstanding. SQUIRE 2.0 provides specific definitions for each term so users will know how the SQUIRE authors intended each term to be interpreted in the guidelines. The website also contains an important explanation and elaboration (E&E) section.[6]

The E&E supports the use of SQUIRE 2.0 by providing representative examples of high-quality reporting of each item, an analysis of each item, and a consideration of the features of the chosen example that are consistent with the item's intent. Each subsubsection of the E&E was peer reviewed and written by a contributing author or authors chosen for their expertise in that area.

In addition to using SQUIRE 2.0 for preparation of articles for health care journals, it is a useful framework for preparing abstracts and posters. Many regional, national, and international conferences accept submissions of improvement work for posters and oral presentations. The SQUIRE 2.0 guidelines provide appropriate headers that can be used in an abstract or on a poster.

# Differentiating Between Improvement and Research

One of the thorny issues that arises in institutions is whether improvement needs to be reviewed by an ethics committee or the Institutional Review Board (IRB). Improvers, researchers, clinicians, and administrators all may be confused about whether proposed work is improvement or research. Laws, regulations, and oversight of research differ from country to country, so we strongly recommend that you learn about the standards of your local ethics committee. The comments in this section pertain to the oversight of research activities in the United States that are administered through the US Department of Health and Human Services Office for Human Research Protections (OHRP) (https://www.hhs.gov/ohrp). A vital first step is determining whether proposed improvement work has any elements of clinical research with human subjects.

IRBs are focused on and comfortable with review and oversight of research projects. These projects use research methodologies to generate new generalizable knowledge and compare differences between groups. Because IRBs may be unfamiliar with the intent and methods used in improvement, the SQUIRE guidelines provide a basis to describe exactly what composes the essential elements and compare these to clinical research with human subjects (*see* Table 9-2 on page 148).[7] This tool consists of four overarching questions and six domains with which to assess

a proposed project: Intent and Background, Methods, Intended Benefit, Risk, Applicability of Results, and Sharing and Disseminating Results. You can use this checklist to assess a proposed project. If there is even *one* check mark in the right-hand column, the project has some element of research and it is appropriate to review the project with the local IRB. If the project only has check marks in the improvement column, then it is acceptable to proceed according to your local institutional oversight and guidance on improvement activities.

The instrument is not intended as an absolute adjudicator between improvement and research with human subjects, but rather as a tool to clarify the components of each. When used well, this instrument provides a means of conversation between improvers, researchers, and IRBs so that patients, staff, and systems are appropriately protected.

## Section Summary

It has been said that "your improvement work is incomplete until it is published."[8] This may not be true for every improvement project, but this certainly should hold true for those who are interested in scholarly improvement work. By sharing improvement—both the successes and failures—in the published literature, we can speed the rate of change and decrease waste in our systems. SQUIRE 2.0 is one tool that provides a common set of criteria that helps in disseminating improvement work.

### Professional education about improvement

*Jennifer and Tomas feel strongly that the ability to improve care should be part of what physicians and nurses (and all health care professionals) learn from the very beginning of their education. Maureen is a 4th grade teacher so also fully understands the need to develop the next generation of health care professionals. They researched literature about education in QI and realized that here was another place they could contribute! Some of the best minds in health professions education agreed with them about the importance of teaching about improvement, but lots of questions remained about how best to do it. Should it be in the classroom or in the clinical setting as part of the usual work flow? After speaking with the associate deans for curriculum in the nursing and medical schools, the team met to discuss what had been learned and how to move forward. Team members learned that the administrators at both schools were very enthusiastic and in need of faculty to lead this interprofessional initiative. Now the three of them wondered, "Where do we start?"*

TABLE 9-2 Instrument to Differentiate Between Quality Improvement and Clinical Research with Human Subjects, Modified Based on SQUIRE 2.0

This table is intended to compare and contrast the general characteristics of quality improvement (QI) and research activities and is for use by Institutional Review Boards (IRBs), QI reviewers, investigators, and improvers. This table is intended to guide discussion among these individuals and is not intended to supplant the judgment of IRBs or QI ethics review committees.

Please start by considering these overarching questions:
1. Will the activities of this project occur within the **standard of care**? If NO, then proceed to IRB review.
2. Is there risk? If YES, use the chart below to determine whether this project requires QI review or IRB review.
3. Is this project primarily intended to generate generalizable knowledge? If YES, proceed to IRB review.
4. Does this project involve **vulnerable populations**? If YES, use the chart below to determine whether this project requires QI review or IRB review.

For each item, choose the column to which the project most closely relates—QI or research. You may choose only one answer. Leave the item blank if neither choice applies.

| Attribute | *Quality Improvement* | *Clinical Research* with Human Subjects |
|---|---|---|
| Intent and Background | ☐ Describes the nature and significance of the local problem. | ☐ Identifies a specific deficit in scientific knowledge from the literature. |
| | ☐ Focus is to improve a specific aspect of health or health care delivery that is currently NOT consistently and appropriately being implemented at this site. | ☐ Proposes to address or identify specific hypotheses in order to develop new knowledge or advance existing knowledge. |
| Methods | ☐ Mechanisms of the intervention are expected to change over time (an iterative activity) in response to ongoing feedback. | ☐ Specific protocol defines the intervention, interaction, and use of collected data and tissues, plus project may rely on the randomization of individuals to enhance confidence in differences. |
| | ☐ Plan for intervention and analysis includes an assessment of the system (process flow diagram, fishbone, etc.) and the context. | ☐ May use qualitative or quantitative methods to make observations, make comparisons between groups, or generate hypotheses. |
| | ☐ Statistical methods evaluate system-level processes and outcomes over time with statistical process control or other methods. | ☐ Statistical methods primarily compare differences between groups or correlate observed differences with a known health condition. |

| TABLE 9-2 | Instrument to Differentiate Between Quality Improvement and Clinical Research with Human Subjects, Modified Based on SQUIRE 2.0 *(continued)* |
|---|---|

| Attribute | *Quality Improvement* | *Clinical Research* with Human Subjects |
|---|---|---|
| **Intended Benefit** | ☐ Intervention would be considered within the usual clinician-patient therapeutic relationship. | ☐ Intervention, interaction, or use of identifiable private information occurs outside of the usual clinician-patient therapeutic relationship. |
| | ☐ Direct benefit to participants is indicated (for example, decrease in risk by receiving a vaccination or by creating a safer institutional system). | ☐ Direct benefit to each individual participant or for the institution is not typically the intent or is not certain. |
| | ☐ Potential local institutional benefit is specified (for example, increased efficiency or decreased cost). | ☐ Potential societal benefit in developing new or advancing existing generalizable knowledge |
| **Risk** | ☐ Primary risk is to privacy or the confidentiality of health information. | ☐ Risks may be minimal, but may include physical, psychological, emotional, social, or financial risks, as well as risk to privacy or the confidentiality of health information from participation in the project. |
| | ☐ Risk may be described as higher for patients by not participating in this activity. | ☐ The informed consent process describes the risks to participants, who individually and voluntarily decide whether to participate, or an IRB grants an alteration or waiver of the consent process. |
| **Applicability of Results** | ☐ Implementation is immediate so that review of results occurs throughout the process and may be used for next QI activity. | ☐ Results and analysis may be delayed or periodic throughout the duration of the project, except to protect patient safety. The results will primarily be used to inform further investigations but may be implemented directly into clinical practice. |
| | ☐ Extrapolation of results to other settings is possible, but not the main *intent* of the activity. | ☐ Results are intended to generalize beyond the study population. |

| TABLE 9-2 | Instrument to Differentiate Between Quality Improvement and Clinical Research with Human Subjects, Modified Based on SQUIRE 2.0 *(continued)* |

| Attribute | *Quality Improvement* | *Clinical Research* with Human Subjects |
|---|---|---|
| **Sharing & Disseminating Results** | ☐ System-level outcomes, processes, refinement of the intervention, and the applicability of the intervention in specific settings/contexts may be shared through peer-reviewed publication and presentation outside the institution. | ☐ It is expected that results will be published or presented to others through a peer-reviewed process. |

SQUIRE, Standards for Quality Improvement Reporting Excellence.

**Interpretation**
Any check marks (even one) in the "Clinical Research" column indicates that there are components of clinical research in the proposed activity. The IRB or QI ethics review mechanism should initiate a discussion with the improver/investigator to clarify the proposal. If an activity such as public health practice, program evaluation, or QI includes a research component, then IRB review should occur under current federal guidance and the policies of many institutions.

**Explanation and Elaboration of Terms**
1. **Standard of Care.** A diagnostic and treatment process that a clinician should follow for a certain type of patient, illness, or clinical circumstance.

2. **Vulnerable population.** Any study population that includes students, employees, children, pregnant women, prisoners, active military personnel, individuals who have impaired decision-making capacity, or those who are educationally or economically disadvantaged.

3. **Intent.** The state of the investigator's mind that directs the activity.

4. **Quality improvement.** The combined and unceasing efforts of everyone—health care professionals, patients and their families, researchers, administrators, payers, planners, educators—to make changes that will lead to better patient outcome, better system performance, and better professional development.

5. **Clinical research.** A systematic investigation in a clinical setting designed to develop or contribute to generalizable knowledge (the Common Rule definition of research).

Ogrinc G, et al. An instrument to differentiate between clinical research and quality improvement. *IRB: Ethics & Human Research.* 2013 Sep–Oct;35(5):1–8. Printed with permission.

# General Principles for Educational Experiences in Health Care Improvement

In the scenario, Jennifer, Tomas, and Maureen were excited about the opportunity to incorporate QI and patient safety into medical and nursing education, but then asked,

"Where do we start?" Four principles for building educational experiences in health care improvement help answer that question. The principles apply to learners at any developmental level. The first three echo what health care educators have found helpful when teaching in other content areas. The fourth arises from what is needed for successful change and improvement in health care.

## Principle 1: The learning experience should be a combination of didactic and project-based work.

Like other complex clinical tasks, learning to improve health care requires mastering new content, acquiring new skills, and demonstrating appropriate attitudes. Thus, there is a need for reading and discussion, reflection, practice, feedback, more discussion, more reflection, more practice, more feedback. This is the classic cycle of experiential learning described by Kolb.[9]

Many of us have learned this lesson the hard way . . . sometimes more than once! One early course in improvement that included medical, nursing, and health administration students at Case Western Reserve University started out with a strong dose of theory, followed by interprofessional student group visits to local health care improvement teams.[10] Each student group's assignment was to learn about the team's project, interview the participants, and report back on how what they had observed illustrated the theory discussed in class. In their feedback about the course, the students strongly endorsed the connection to real-time health care improvement work, but like health professions students everywhere, they wanted to participate, not just observe. (We know what you're thinking: This point does seem obvious now!) The next time the university offered the course, interprofessional student teams worked on projects sponsored by local health care improvement leaders, usually carved out from larger initiatives. The course faculty prepared the students with several weeks of didactic work before the projects began. Student feedback was more positive than before, but the students felt strongly that they would learn more by going to work on their projects as soon as possible.

By the time the course reached a steady-state model (with consistently high ratings from both the students and the project sponsors), the students signed up for their projects as part of signing up for the course, had their first student team meeting during the first class, and started on their projects right away. Didactic work in class supported the project work, not the other way around. Student learning, as measured by the quality of project reports, improved. Project sponsors returned to offer student projects year after year. Even teams made up of novice health professions students contributed to health care improvement projects in ways that were valuable to the host organizations.

This leads to two corollary principles:
1. Didactic learning seems to "stick" best when it is related to project work.
2. The most stimulating projects are those that are most likely to create a direct benefit to patients.

All of this echoes what generations of learners have said—that learning in the context of real patient problems is most stimulating and most likely to be retained over time.[11]

## Principle 2: Link with health system improvement efforts.

A long-standing (and not yet resolved) controversy among health care improvement teachers is the value of learner-initiated improvement projects. The argument is compelling: Learners will be most stimulated to work on (and learn from) projects they have identified themselves and in which they have a particular interest. The problem is that what learners wish to improve may not align with the top priorities of health care organizations and their leaders. In that case, progress may occur only as long as the learner-champion keeps the work going. When the inevitable occurs and the learner moves on to another course, another clerkship, another rotation, another training program, work on the project may end then and there. That is often before significant improvements have occurred, even with the best learner efforts and ideas. That final result can be frustrating for both students and faculty. The better approach is to align improvement learning with actual clinical projects.[12–14] We suggest two ways to deal with this dilemma: (1) carefully prepare the learner-initiated project before the learner gets started or (2) invite the learner to choose from a menu of projects created from a list of current organizational priorities.

### Carefully prepare the learner-initiated project before the learner gets started.

To prepare for a successful learner-initiated improvement project, it is important to ask who must support the work for anything new to happen. What part of the organization is involved? Who are the leaders? Whose support will be needed for change to occur? Who will be the project champion (and team) after the learner moves on? It is a good idea to talk with those people before any work starts and enlist their help; ideally, you want to recruit them to be part of the improvement team. Consider the triangle in Figure 9-1 on page 152. In any health care organization, improved patient outcomes and system performance will be as important as excellent professional development.[15] Who needs to be involved and what will it take to be sure that the learner-initiated project resonates in all three areas?

FIGURE 9-1

## Batalden and Davidoff's Definition of Quality Improvement in Health Care

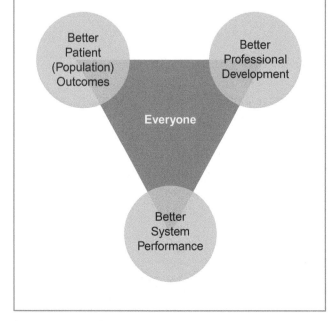

**Source:** Batalden PB, Davidoff F. What is "quality improvement" and how can it transform healthcare? *Qual Saf Health Care*. 2007 Feb;16(1):2–3. Reprinted with permission from the BMJ Publishing Group Limited.

An example of preparation for a successful learner-initiated improvement project is a project done by a medical resident to decrease the rate of central line–associated infections in the medical intensive care unit (MICU) through more reliable use of full-barrier protection (that is, sterile drapes, gown, gloves, mask) during line insertion. The resident was passionate about the project, but his success depended on partnerships with leaders in the MICU who had the authority to make things happen. In this case, a key partner was the nurse unit manager, who worked with the resident to test the intervention(s) (including a procedure cart with all the necessary materials easily at hand) and to sustain its use over time (after the resident finished his part of the project and moved on to another rotation). Without these steps, learners may become very frustrated at not being able to get anything done or, even with a successful project, having no way to sustain improvements when they must inevitably move on to other assignments.

A common and widely used assignment for senior nursing students is to identify and execute a QI project during their cumulative clinical capstone course. Having learners work closely with unit managers in identifying these projects creates mutual benefit for the senior nursing student and the nursing unit. The nursing literature is replete with examples of such projects.[16–19]

### Invite the learner to choose from a menu of projects created from a list of current organizational priorities.

An alternate approach to preparing for a successful learner-initiated improvement project is to identify health care improvement efforts that are already in place and thus already have gained the support and investment of the organization's leaders. It is often not difficult to identify a part of that work that could benefit from another set of willing hands. It is challenging to have learners become part of ongoing project teams; the rhythm of a learner's life usually does not match the work cycle of an ongoing improvement team. Despite the best intentions on all sides, the learner may rarely be able to attend routinely scheduled meetings. Instead, if someone from the improvement team is willing to act as a project sponsor, learners can often take over a certain area (think of it as a "subproject"), work on it during the time available to meet prespecified goals, and then hand it back to the team. An example is an organizational effort to improve the care of patients with sickle cell disease. The team identified multiple issues that led to patients with severe sickle cell disease receiving most of their care in the emergency department. While the team worked on improving the organization's approach to managing pain with sickle cell crises, a learner team worked to identify the barriers to clinic follow-up after observing a sickle cell patient's experience in the emergency room. The learners interviewed the patients to understand the issues from the patients' point of view and made several recommendations that the team later tested.

## Principle 3: Assess education outcomes.

As part of an outstanding review of interprofessional education, Hugh Barr and colleagues created a helpful elaboration of the classic Kirkpatrick model of education outcomes. We reprint it in Table 9-3 on page 153, along with an example of the model's application in improvement education.[20] Barr et al.'s work was published two years before Batalden and Davidoff published Figure 9-1,[15] yet the similarities are striking. Perhaps we shouldn't be surprised, as improvement work at its core is about

## TABLE 9-3   Barr-Kirkpatrick Hierarchy of Educational Outcomes

| Education Outcome | Example |
|---|---|
| 1. Reaction | End-of-experience student feedback |
| 2a. Modification of attitudes/perceptions | Pre- and post-student responses to written assessment of attitudes related to health care quality, patient safety, and interprofessional teamwork |
| 2b. Acquisition of knowledge/skills | Assessment of ability to read a case scenario, identify an improvement need, write an aim statement, identify an appropriate measure, and propose a change to test |
| 3. Behavioral change | During a clinical rotation, 360-degree assessment of behaviors consistent with collaboration and teamwork |
| 4a. Change in organizational practice | Change in care as a result of an improvement initiative |
| 4b. Benefits to patients/clients | Change in patient outcomes related to an improvement initiative |

**Source:** Barr H, et al. *Effective Interprofessional Education—Argument, Assumption and Evidence.* Oxford, UK: Blackwell, 2005. Printed with permission.

learning. It is impressive that Barr and colleagues identified change in organizational practice and benefits to patients as the highest order of education outcomes.

The model starts with the most commonly used education outcome—learner feedback. Learner feedback is critical to improving the quality of a learning experience, but when used alone, it can be misleading. In one example, medical residents who experienced (and liked) a popular classroom-based introduction to improvement performed no better than controls when a written knowledge application assessment tested their improvement learning.[21] In contrast, medical residents who underwent a course involving a combination of a health care improvement project and didactics performed much better than controls on a similar instrument.[12] Although both groups of residents rated their learning experiences highly, they performed much differently when their ability to apply what they learned was assessed.

Education about QI in health care creates opportunities for educators to link their efforts to improvements in patient outcomes and organizational performance, the other end of Barr's outcomes typology. Some have succeeded in doing just that, even with inexperienced learners.[13,14,22,23] We suggest that teachers creating learning experiences in health care improvement focus on a few key outcome measures (from as many levels of Barr's model you can manage) and work to collect those in a way that will give feedback to both the learners and the teachers. Two helpful questions might be "What is the single most important attribute I'm trying to engender in these learners?" and "How can I measure that in a way that will be useful?"

## Principle 4: Role-model QI in educational processes.

Education outcomes have a dual purpose: feedback for the learner and feedback for the teacher. We believe that part of the work of teaching improvement is modeling the same improvement behaviors in our work as educators. Why would learners believe that QI is important, if they don't see the faculty improving their own work, both as clinicians and educators?

In the published examples described in the text, the faculty received important information about education outcomes through surveys to collect learner feedback, written tests of learner ability to apply knowledge, structured assessments of learner team project reports, organization sponsor feedback, and changes in organizational practice and patient outcomes. Any and all of these can be used to improve a learning experience, applying QI to education itself. We need to be sure to schedule time to reflect on the results of our education efforts and make decisions about the future. When the teaching is over and the learner feedback given, it's easy to move on to the next agenda item in our busy professional lives. QI depends on reflection (the "Act" phase of the PDSA cycle described in Chapter 7), without which our efforts will fail to improve over time.

# Health Professional Development in the Improvement of Health Care Quality

We've already referenced Batalden and Davidoff's classic 2007 editorial, in which they asked "What is 'quality improvement' and how can it transform healthcare?"[15] They wrote that QI is "the combined and unceasing efforts of everyone—healthcare professionals, patients and their families, researchers, payers, planners, and educators—to make the changes that will lead to better patient outcomes (health), better system performance (care) and better professional development (learning)"[15(p. 2)] (*see* Figure 9-1). In the opening scenario of this chapter, Jennifer, Maureen, and Tomas's experience with the RRT is an excellent example of such efforts. How can we systematically ensure that everyone is using QI to make changes that will lead to better outcomes and performance?

In a 2003 follow-up to the landmark report *Crossing the Quality Chasm*,[24] the Institute of Medicine (IOM) convened an interprofessional panel to consider the implications for health professions education. As a result, the IOM advocated that all learners and working health professionals develop and maintain proficiency in delivering patient-centered care, working as part of interdisciplinary teams, practicing evidence-based medicine, focusing on QI, and using information technology.[25] QI is an increasingly visible aspect of clinical practice, but such work will not become "business as usual" until training in essential improvement skills is built into every level of health professional preparation.

Accordingly, educational and accrediting organizations across the health professions recognize the need for knowledge, skills, and attitudes that prepare learners to participate in improvement. Nursing created Quality and Safety Education for Nurses (QSEN), a vibrant community offering resources and models for nursing education (http://www.qsen.org). In medical education, the Accreditation Council for Graduate Medical Education (ACGME) made improvement an essential part of physician professional responsibility, establishing "practice-based learning and improvement" and "systems-based practice" as two of six core competencies required in all postgraduate training programs.[26] Similarly, the Association of American Medical Colleges wrote in its Teaching for Quality report that "quality improvement is core to what it means to be a physician."[27(p. 23)] Other health care disciplines also expect competencies related to system improvement to be included in professional curricula, including the Accreditation Review Commission on Education for the Physician Assistant (http://www.arc-pa.org), the Accreditation Council for Pharmacy Education (https://www.acpe-accredit.org), and the Commission on Dental Accreditation (http://www.ada.org/en/coda).

The overlap and commonalities among the health professions are striking. Although different health professions have organized their competencies and requirements in different ways (for example, ACGME focuses on practice-based learning and improvement and systems-based practice, while QSEN focuses on QI and safety), each builds on the recommendations of the 2003 IOM report, creating a framework for both educators and learners to use in developing professional competency.

## Competency in Quality Improvement

Why do many accreditation organizations use the term *competency*? Why not use *skills*—or even *domains of learning*? The term *competency* is useful because it links stages of professional development with general models of adult learning. Although individuals acquire and assimilate knowledge and skills in different ways, an appreciation of general developmental stages permits both learners and educators (including instructors, mentors, and coaches) to create and structure optimal learning experiences.

In the 1970s Hubert and Stewart Dreyfus, focusing on chess players and pilots, described five stages (and characteristics) of skill development: novice, advanced beginner, competent, proficient, and expert.[28] Because health professionals are expected to achieve a level of competence by the end of training, health professions educators must understand the experience of learners in each of the Dreyfus stages. In the 1980s nursing theorist Patricia Benner used the Dreyfus stages to articulate levels of clinical growth and development in expert nurse clinicians.[29] Benner's work has been foundational in bringing the Dreyfus model to health professions education.

Health care improvement is not a "spectator sport" but a participant-driven implementation of specific knowledge and skills. Health professionals cannot learn to make such improvements by sitting passively in a lecture, attending a meeting, or visiting a website, although websites, didactic sessions, and other materials can play an important role in preparing the learner. Improvement is an action, thus learning about improvement must be action based. But what skills and knowledge are required at each stage in this learning process so health professional learners achieve competence in QI before entering practice? Let us more closely examine each stage in the Dreyfus model of professional development and identify specific improvement-oriented educational strategies at each.

- **Novice:** At the novice level, learners attend to basic rules rather than to the real-world application of these rules. (In the spirit of *Dragnet*, novices want "just the facts.") Instructors, in turn, must make these rules the focus of their educational efforts. Knowledge at this level is free of context, and as a result, learners' simple application of such rules may produce poor results in the real world. Novices need to learn basic knowledge, skills, tools, and techniques for improvement, so they benefit from a source of core knowledge such as the information in this book; however, experiential learning is also essential.

*For example, learners begin to gain knowledge about health care systems by working within an interprofessional team (with other novices). They may learn about QI in small-group or lecture settings (supplemented by readings) and by carrying out specific assigned tasks. Novices can take part in activities such as interviewing key stakeholders to validate a draft fishbone diagram. Another strategy is to involve learners in specific aspects of improvement work that enables them to contribute fresh insights that might be missed by more senior clinicians who are immersed every day in the (dys)functions of the health care system. For instance, a learner following a patient being admitted to the hospital from the emergency department can describe the steps of that process from the*

*patient's point of view, identifying areas for possible improvement.*

- **Advanced Beginner:** As the novice gains initial experience with real situations, he or she progresses to the next level. Experience interacts with and contextualizes the rules, and the nature of the interaction becomes important. This "work in context" enhances basic knowledge and skills. The advanced beginner needs opportunities to apply rules "in action," which provide important experiences in multiple places/contexts. Such opportunities may be constructed around formal QI rotations or QI experiences embedded within other coursework or clinical rotations. These multiple contexts enable learners to participate in and realize the benefits of interprofessional learning in action, specifically through collaboration with learners across disciplines.

*The advanced beginner needs to apply improvement concepts and tools to real-world situations. One example is to review publicly available data on the quality of care at the hospital in which he or she will be working. Two great resources for this are the Hospital Compare website (https://www.medicare.gov/hospitalcompare/search.html) and The Joint Commission's Quality Check® (https://www.qualitycheck.org). Learners can explore these websites to identify priorities for improving patient outcomes. The learners can sketch out a QI project focusing on the identified priorities. In examining patterns and trends of QI data, the learner can recognize the importance of variation in understanding QI process outcomes. Ideally, educators place learners on an improvement team within the facility during their clinical training. For example, an advanced beginner—primed with the foundational knowledge and skills from learning as a novice—can walk the team through the process of working to improve vaccination rates in clinic. The learner can prepare the first draft of a flow diagram that forms the foundation for the team to discuss the process. As the learner gains QI experience in many settings, he or she progresses through the advanced beginner stage.*

- **Competent:** The learner becomes competent in improvement when he or she can use QI methods to assess a system, use data to monitor quality and safety outcomes of the new process, and design and test changes. Competence occurs after a great deal of experience. Learners begin to appreciate which elements of the situation require attention and which do not. The vast possibilities of interpretation or action can be narrowed to a manageable few. In addition, competence includes a deeper emotional attachment to the work. The learner "owns" the process and feels the joys and disappointments when the work is successful or not.

As discussed earlier in this chapter, accreditation agencies have set competence as the level required for independent practice, so this level is essential for practicing professionals. Knowledge of QI and safety is part of the licensure exam for new registered nurses from the National Council of State Boards of Nursing (https://www.ncsbn.org/nclex.htm). Physicians in all member specialties must demonstrate that they can assess the quality of care they provide compared to peers and national benchmarks and then apply the best evidence or consensus recommendations to improve that care using follow-up assessments (American Board of Medical Specialties; http://www.abms.org).

Competence in QI implies independent ability for individuals who are ready, willing, and able to engage in, role-model, and fully participate in improvement work. Often this is through leading or coleading QI work. They identify patient and system outcomes that need improvement and can initiate PDSA cycles. Competence in improvement usually develops near the end of formal professional training and the beginning of the professional career.

*A new staff nurse, a third-year internal medicine resident, and a pharmacy intern notice that there is no coordination for discharging patients from the hospital who take warfarin, an oral blood thinner. The three meet to discuss and, using their QI skills developed throughout their training, start by bringing a team together that includes a patient recently discharged from the hospital on warfarin. Under the coaching of the hospital QI leader, they facilitate writing a clear aim, map the process of discharge and follow-up for warfarin, identify and analyze data, and begin to test changes to the system. These three lead the team through the improvement work, relying on each other and their QI coach when they get stuck or need direction. The culmination of all their QI learning through professional school and postgraduate training has made them comfortable leading and participating in QI work.*

- **Proficient:** This stage is an extension of competence and is achieved after being involved in many levels of improvement work over time. Proficient practitioners take waste out of the work. The proficient individual continues to scroll through a list of possibilities for the work and does so with much greater speed. An element

of *efficiency* now accompanies the work. Individuals can step back and more clearly see the problem that needs to be solved, though often the solution itself still requires active deliberation. Increased efficiency enables the practitioner to remove waste from the work by directly connecting knowledge and skill to the problem at hand. The proficient QI professional may use advanced QI assessment and measurement methods and knows when to call on these advanced methods. The proficient QI professional easily leads QI teams and may serve as a peer coach for other QI team leaders. Often this level also involves teaching QI knowledge and skills to others and may include presenting QI work at academic meetings and publishing that work in peer-reviewed health care literature.

Those who become proficient in QI may seek out additional training through a certificate program, graduate degree, or profession- or specialty-specific training to develop their skills. Over the past two decades, increasing numbers of certificate programs, graduate programs, and postgraduate training programs are focused on quality and safety. The growing number of programs speaks to the increased need within the larger health care system for professionals with advanced QI and safety knowledge and skills.

*A junior medicine faculty member had several experiences in her physician residency program applying QI knowledge and skills and seeing improved, evidence-based care for patients. She is now facile at leading QI teams and regularly confers with other QI team leaders in the hospital, creating a peer network to learn together. She works to incorporate improvement into routine practice and includes QI and safety as part of her teaching. However, she desires a greater depth of knowledge and skills in QI, so she enrolls in a specialty-specific course about leading and teaching QI. While enrolled in this certificate program, she collaborates with an administrator, a physical therapist, and a patient representative to write an abstract (using the SQUIRE 2.0 guidelines) for a national conference about their home-based physical therapy program, which has improved function for patients and decreased costs for the system. She is a little uncertain about this process, but excited about the prospect of sharing the team's good work with others.*

- **Expert:** The expert develops a vast repertoire of skills and a capacity for situational discrimination that are achievable only through substantial experience. He or she can perform tasks on a more intuitive level and recognize and immediately address essential problems. Experts in QI learn to manage situations in which the rules do not apply or adapt methods to meet the needs of unusual problems. Experts relish the unusual and challenging problems that arise. They are recognized locally as "go-to" persons in improvement and may also take on leadership roles in clinical and/or professional organizations to improve outcomes within the health care system. Experts often study the improvement work and regularly seek to publish and present their work. Developing expertise in QI is a personal commitment to do so and can occur only with substantial improvement experiences and ongoing professional development over time.

*An assistant professor in the College of Nursing completes a two-year interprofessional fellowship in Quality and Safety, learning advanced process modeling techniques and analysis tools such as statistical process control for monitoring changes of infrequent events. His new skills make him the point person for the tough QI problems in the institution where he is known as a QI leader and mentor for others. He works with other local QI experts to develop a new interprofessional master's degree in Quality and Safety at the university. Using the Barr-Kirkpatrick model, the team of experts evaluates the outcomes of the degree program, including the impact on quality and safety indicators at the academic health system. This team is regularly invited to speak and consult with others about developing an improvement culture in other health care organizations.*

In adapting the developmental language of the Dreyfus model to the specific challenges of health professions training in QI, educators can recognize that training is a process of ongoing professional growth and development. Acquisition of specific knowledge and skills is essential for all professionals, but terms such as *competent* and *proficient* direct our attention to practitioners' underlying capacity to *assimilate* and *apply* their knowledge and skills—with increasing sophistication. In the work of health care improvement, competence must mature and develop over time similar to other professional knowledge and skills.

## Summary

To ensure safe, high-quality care, it is important for health professional learners and practitioners to have knowledge and skills for improvement work. The knowledge and skills should be embedded early in health professions curricula and need to include project-based work within

interprofessional teams ideally "across the street" within the walls of the school's clinical partners. In keeping with the spirit of improvement, these teaching strategies should be evaluated for effectiveness beyond learner reaction and skills assessment; they should also be evaluated by looking at change in organizational practice and benefits to patients. This organized approach to professional development can guide more health professionals from novice to competent/ proficient improvement practitioners who will lead initiatives to improve system performance and patient outcomes that can transform health care.

## References

1.  Davidoff F, et al. Publication guidelines for quality improvement in healthcare: Evolution of the SQUIRE project. *Qual Saf Health Care*. 2008 Oct;17 Suppl 1::i3–9.
2.  Ogrinc G, et al. SQUIRE 2.0 (Standards for Quality Improvement Reporting Excellence): Revised publication guidelines from a detailed consensus process. *BMJ Qual Saf*. 2016 Dec;25(12):986–992.
3.  Davidoff F, et al. Demystifying theory and its use in improvement. *BMJ Qual Saf*. 2015 Mar;24(3):228–238.
4.  Rycroft-Malone J. The PARIHS framework—A framework for guiding the implementation of evidence-based practice. *J Nurs Care Qual*. 2004 Oct–Dec;19(4):297–304.
5.  Damschroder L, et al. Fostering implementation of health services research findings into practice: A consolidated framework for advancing implementation science. *Implement Sci*. 2009 Aug 7;4:50.
6.  Goodman D, et al. Explanation and elaboration of the SQUIRE (Standards for Quality Improvement Reporting Excellence) Guidelines, V.2.0: Examples of SQUIRE elements in the healthcare improvement literature. *BMJ Qual Saf*. 2016 Dec;25(12):e7.
7.  Ogrinc G, et al. An instrument to differentiate between clinical research and quality improvement. *IRB: Ethics & Human Research*. 2013 Sep–Oct;35(5):1–8.
8.  Stevens DP, Marshall BC. Healthcare improvement is incomplete until it is published: The cystic fibrosis initiative to support scholarly publication. *BMJ Qual Saf*. 2014 Apr;23 Suppl 1:i104–107.
9.  Kolb DA. *Experiential Learning: Experience as the Source of Learning and Development*. Englewood Cliffs, NJ: Prentice-Hall, 1984.
10. Moore SM, et al. Using learning cycles to build an interdisciplinary curriculum in CI for health professions students in Cleveland. *Jt Comm J Qual Improv*. 1996 Mar;22(3):165–171.

11. Hoffman K, et al. Problem-based learning outcomes: Ten years of experience at the University of Missouri–Columbia School of Medicine. *Acad Med*. 2006 Jul;81(7):617–625.

12. Ogrinc G, et al. Teaching and assessing resident competence in practice-based learning and improvement. *J Gen Intern Med*. 2004 May;19(5 Pt 2):496–500.

13. Hall L, et al. Linking health professional learners and healthcare workers on action-based improvement teams. *Qual Manag Health Care*. 2009 Jul–Sep;18(3):194–201.

14. Ogrinc G, et al. Clinical and educational outcomes of an integrated inpatient quality improvement curriculum for internal medicine residents. *J Grad Med Educ*. 2016 Oct;8(4):563–568.

15. Batalden PB, Davidoff F. What is "quality improvement" and how can it transform healthcare? *Qual Saf Health Care*. 2007 Feb;16(1):2–3.

16. Baillie L, et al. Implementing service improvement projects within pre-registration nursing education: A multi-method case study evaluation. *Nurse Educ Pract*. 2014 Jan;14(1):62–68.

17. Crist JD, et al. Addressing future demands: Nursing students, elders, and pet birds: A student-initiated quality improvement project. *Geriatr Nurs*. 2017 Mar–Apr;38(2):160–164.

18. James B, et al. Time, fear and transformation: Student nurses' experiences of doing a practicum (quality improvement project) in practice. *Nurse Educ Pract*. 2016 Jul;19:70–78.

19. Tschannen D, et al. Improving patient care through student leadership in team quality improvement projects. *J Nurs Care Qual*. 2015 Apr–Jun;30(2):181–186.

20. Barr H, et al. Effective Interprofessional Education—Argument, Assumption and Evidence. Oxford, UK: Blackwell, 2005.

21. Morrison LJ, Headrick LA. Teaching residents about practice-based learning and improvement. *Jt Comm J Qual Patient Saf*. 2008 Aug;34(8):453–459.

22. Gould BE et al. Improving patient care outcomes by teaching quality improvement to medical students in community-based practices. *Acad Med*. 2002 Oct;77(10):1011–1018.

23. Hall LW, et al. Effectiveness of patient safety training in equipping medical students to recognise safety hazards and propose robust interventions. *Qual Saf Health Care*. 2010 Feb;19(1):3–8.

24. Institute of Medicine. *Crossing the Quality Chasm: A New Health System for the 21st Century*. Washington, DC: National Academy Press, 2001.

25. Institute of Medicine. *Health Professions Education: A Bridge to Quality*. Washington, DC: National Academies Press; 2003.

26. Batalden P, et al. General competencies and accreditation in graduate medical education. *Health Aff* (Millwood). 2002 Sep–Oct;21(5):103–111.

27. Headrick LA, et al. *Teaching for Quality: Integrating Quality Improvement and Patient Safety Across the Continuum of Medical Education: Report of an Expert Panel*. Washington, DC: Association of American Medical Colleges, 2013. Accessed Nov 26, 2017. https://www.aamc.org/initiatives/cei/te4q/366184/te4qreportarticle.html.

28. Dreyfus H, Dreyfus S. *Mind over Machine: The Power of Human Intuition and Expertise in the Era of the Computer*. New York: Free Press, 1986.

29. Benner P. *From Novice to Expert: Excellence and Power in Clinical Nursing Practice*. Upper Saddle River, NJ: Prentice Hall, 1984.

# Appendix: Tools to Help Your Improvement

This appendix contains 16 tools that can be useful for doing and teaching improvement. The authors compiled these tools in an educational program offered through Case Western Reserve University and the Institute for Healthcare Improvement. They range from an improvement project worksheet (that aligns with the content in this book) to meeting processes to time lines to Plan–Do–Study–Act (PDSA) worksheets. Some tools (for example, the process map, fishbone diagram, and PDSA worksheet) augment and supplement material presented in this book. Other tools (for example, developing a survey and collecting data and team evaluation) provide tips for additional skills.

The tools provided in this appendix are not intended as comprehensive instructions but rather as useful supplements with which to get started. Table A-0 (page 160) lists each tool and the page on which it can be found.

## Improvement Project Worksheet

This two-sided worksheet was created as a way to "see" and appreciate the overall quality improvement process (*see* Figure A-1, page 161). It consists of a seven-step process that begins with identifying an aim and gathering a team and ends with testing a change intervention with the PDSA cycle.

The seven steps correspond to the following chapters in this book:

       Step 1. Chapter 3
       Step 2. Chapter 2
       Step 3. Chapter 4
       Step 4. Chapter 7
       Step 5. Chapters 5 and 6
       Step 6. Chapter 7
       Step 7. Chapter 7

## The Seven-Step Meeting Process

The seven-step meeting process allows your team to maximize the time you spend together. The work is divided as follows:

    Steps 1–3:    Warm up, prepare for work.
    Step 4:    Do the work.
    Steps 5–7:    Prepare for next time.

1. Assign roles:
   - Identify roles: Leader, Recorder, Timekeeper, Facilitator.

2. Clarify the objective:
   - Develop and distribute agenda.
   - Bring necessary supplies to the meeting.
   - Establish process/rule for making decisions.
   - Set or review ground rules.

3. Review the agenda:
   - Amend agenda as necessary per team's recommendations.
   - Enhance meeting efficiency with a "timed" agenda.

4. Work through the agenda items:
   - Cover one item at a time.
   - Manage discussions and maintain focus and pace.
   - Solicit team participation.
   - Clarify ambiguous points.
   - Resolve any conflicts.
   - Create a "parking lot" for issues you don't want to address but want to track.

| TABLE A-0 | Summary and Location of Improvement Tools Presented in the Appendix* | |
|---|---|---|

| Tool Name | Purpose | Pages |
|---|---|---|
| Improvement Project Worksheet | Overview of the steps in the improvement process | 159 |
| The Seven-Step Meeting Process | Method to run an efficient and effective meeting | 159 |
| Team Roles | Tool to assist with clarity of roles on a team | 162 |
| Team Charter | Tool to assist with clarification of goal and roles of the team | 163 |
| Readiness for Change | Tool to collect information on the readiness for a unit to engage in improvement work | 164 |
| Stakeholder Assessment | Tool to assess the perspectives of the identified stakeholders | 166 |
| Complex Adaptive System | Tool to understand the complexity of the systems in which improvement work occurs | 166 |
| Time Line | Tool to facilitate the development of a time line to guide the improvement work | 168 |
| Communication Plan | Tool to facilitate communication among team members and stakeholders | 168 |
| Flowchart or Process Map | Tool to assist in the development of a process map | 171 |
| Cause-and-Effect Diagram | Tool to assist in the development of a fishbone diagram | 171 |
| Tips for Developing a Survey and Collecting Real-Time Data | Tips to develop a survey to collect data from frontline workers or stakeholders | 173 |
| Change Concepts Worksheet | Worksheet to identify important change strategies to test in the improvement work | 175 |
| Plan–Do–Study–Act (PDSA) Worksheet | Worksheet to guide small experiments of change | 176 |
| Team Evaluation | GRPI tool to assist in assessing team function | 176 |
| Creating a Storyboard | Guidance and an example to assist with the development of a storyboard | 176 |

* The original tools and worksheets that appear throughout this appendix were compiled by the authors from the following sources and have been used with permission:
1. Dolansky MA, Singh MK, Neuhauser DB. Quality and safety education: Foreground and background, *Qual Manag Health Care*. 2009 Jul–Sep;18(3):151–157.
2. Coursera. Take the Lead on Quality Improvement in Healthcare. Dolansky MA, et al. 2017. Massive Open Online Course. Accessed 27, 2017. https://www.coursera.org/learn/hcqualityimprovement.

**FIGURE A-1** Improvement Project Worksheet

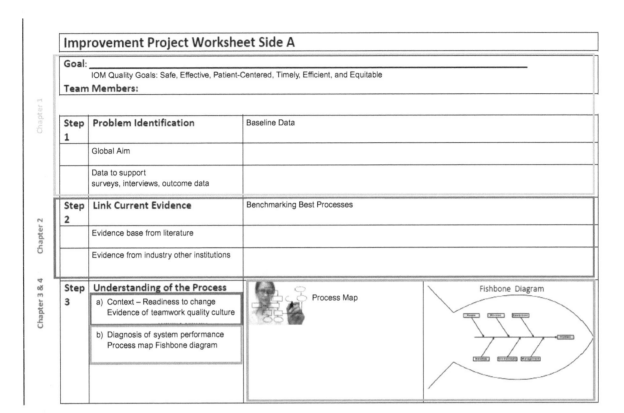

IOM, Institute of Medicine.    IHI, Institute for Healthcare Improvement. Used with permission.

5. Summarize the content of the meeting:
   - Summarize decisions.
   - Review action items.
   - Identify follow-up.
   - Summarize responsibilities of team members.

6. Develop the agenda for the next meeting:
   - Solicit agenda items for next meeting.
   - Review time and place for next meeting.

7. Evaluate the meeting:
   - Identify what went well.
   - Identify what can be improved.
   - Address any remaining questions.

# Team Roles

While each quality improvement (QI) team is unique, there are several roles that most could benefit from, particularly during meetings.

1. **Team Leader**
   Coordinates and directs the work of the team. Manages the work of the team and the process of team meetings.
2. **Recorder**
   Responsible for creating the meeting record. Often it is useful to keep notes on a flip chart, immediately available to everyone (including latecomers). Role usually rotated, meeting to meeting, to share the burden.
3. **Timekeeper**
   Watches the time and alerts the group when the time allotted for a particular agenda item is nearly gone. The timekeeper's role is only to inform; it is up to the team as a whole to decide how to use its time, perhaps revising the agenda to accommodate an agenda item that needs more time than expected.
4. **Facilitator**
   Responsible for keeping the meeting focused and moving smoothly. Identifies members who are not speaking enough or speaking too much.
5. **Team Members**
   Everyone shares responsibility for the work of the team: sharing knowledge and expertise, participating in decision making, using good discussion and listening skills, performing special tasks between meetings as agreed.

# Team Charter

A team charter is a document that is developed by the team to clarify the direction of the project while establishing accountability and boundaries (*see* Table A-1, below). The team charter serves as a source to describe the focus and direction of the team, and it serves to educate others about the team and project.

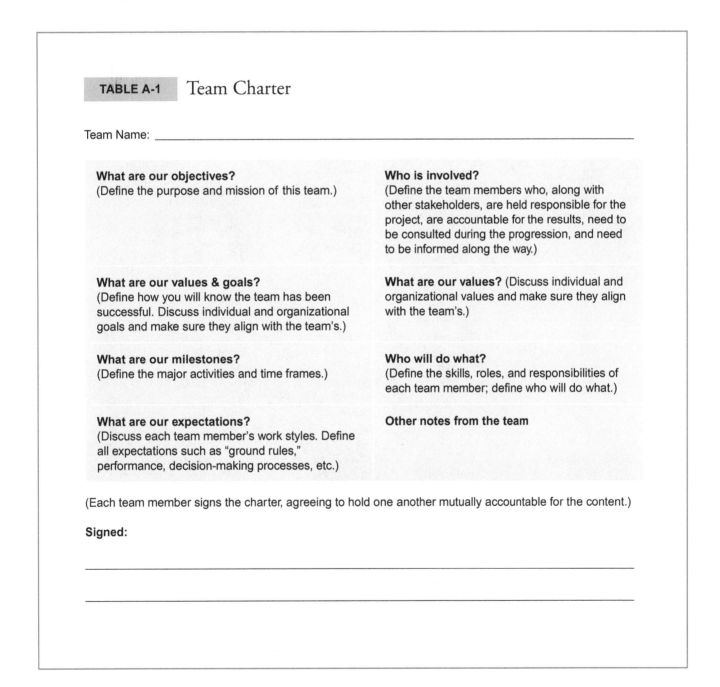

**TABLE A-1**   Team Charter

Team Name: _____

**What are our objectives?**
(Define the purpose and mission of this team.)

**Who is involved?**
(Define the team members who, along with other stakeholders, are held responsible for the project, are accountable for the results, need to be consulted during the progression, and need to be informed along the way.)

**What are our values & goals?**
(Define how you will know the team has been successful. Discuss individual and organizational goals and make sure they align with the team's.)

**What are our values?** (Discuss individual and organizational values and make sure they align with the team's.)

**What are our milestones?**
(Define the major activities and time frames.)

**Who will do what?**
(Define the skills, roles, and responsibilities of each team member; define who will do what.)

**What are our expectations?**
(Discuss each team member's work styles. Define all expectations such as "ground rules," performance, decision-making processes, etc.)

**Other notes from the team**

(Each team member signs the charter, agreeing to hold one another mutually accountable for the content.)

**Signed:**

_____

_____

# Readiness for Change

Table A-2, below, provides a way for teams to understand the attitudes in the unit in which the change will take place. It can be filled out as a worksheet by a unit leader or by multiple staff members and then aggregated to form an average score.

**TABLE A-2**  Readiness for Change

| | Characteristic | Degree of Readiness | | | |
|---|---|---|---|---|---|
| | | **Cold** | **Warm** | **Hot** | **Not sure** |
| 1 | Unit History of Successful QI | ☐ Hmmm . . . where is quality around here? | ☐ Well, I see quality posters on the wall, and the manager talks about quality indicators. Not sure about success. | ☐ I am aware of past successful quality projects on our unit. | ☐ |
| 2 | Need for Change on Unit | ☐ I am not sure what projects we are working on. | ☐ Our unit only works on large institutionwide quality projects that are led by the quality department. | ☐ I am aware of what we need to work on to improve quality on my unit. | ☐ |
| 3 | Priority of Change | ☐ Only Joint Commission projects are talked about. | ☐ It seems a lot of things are going on, but I'm not sure of priorities. | ☐ Our manager makes it clear what projects are high priority and why. Quality projects align with my organization's goals | ☐ |
| 4 | Leadership Support | ☐ We have no time for this—we are too busy giving care. | ☐ Leadership provides me time to improve quality, and I am encouraged to work on quality committees. | ☐ Leadership provides me time and resources to improve quality. | ☐ |

FUNDAMENTALS OF HEALTH CARE IMPROVEMENT  ✿  THIRD EDITION

| | Characteristic | Degree of Readiness | | | |
|---|---|---|---|---|---|
| | | **Cold** | **Warm** | **Hot** | **Not sure** |
| 5 | Staff Support | ☐ No one would want to work with me to improve care. | ☐ I might be able to find some other nurses who would work with me on a project. | ☐ Other nurses are eager to participate in quality projects. | ☐ |
| 6 | Unit Quality Culture | ☐ I don't think it is really important to be involved in quality projects. | ☐ Quality seems to be important on our unit, but I only see the manager and educator working on projects. | ☐ I have tools to help me make changes. Nurses are involved in unit and organizational projects. I feel enthusiasm here. | ☐ |
| 7 | Available Data to Monitor Progress | ☐ I don't know about any data on our unit regarding quality. | ☐ The manager tells us about our data, but I am not sure how to get them or use them. | ☐ Data are available for me to use, and I know how to get them and use them. | ☐ |
| 8 | Interprofessional Team | ☐ I work independently and am responsible for my own part. | ☐ Our work is interprofessional, but we are not always able to work in effective teams. | ☐ The approach is interprofessional. We get secretaries, physicians, and therapists working together. | ☐ |

**Source:** Adapted from Shea C.M, et al. Organizational readiness for implementing change: A psychometric assessment of a new measure. *Implement Sci.* 2014 Jan 10;9:7.
QI, quality improvement.

# Stakeholder Assessment

Stakeholder identification and management are critical tasks in any quality improvement (QI) project. Required elements of planning include identification of key stakeholders, who then either need to be informed or be involved in the project. Table A-3 on page 167 is one sample stakeholder analysis matrix.

## Stakeholders

Any individual or group that is influenced in some way by your proposed project, or in turn can influence the success of your project, is a stakeholder. It is essential that all important stakeholders be identified before the project is implemented, and a decision made as to whether to include them in the project or just keep them informed of the project and how it is progressing. For example, a project to improve any specific type of infection rate needs to include the infection control department. A project to reduce medication errors needs to include pharmacy as well as risk management. Failure to inform or include a key stakeholder might result in your project being stalled or canceled entirely.

Stakeholders can be classified according to anticipated support for your project (support, neutral, oppose) and level of influence in the organization (high, neutral, low). Stakeholders who are likely to oppose the project and have high levels of influence in the organization require the careful planning of strategies to reduce or manage their opposition. Strategies might include early notification about the project and the underlying rationale, use of an influential ally to maintain communication between the implementation team and the stakeholder, or an invitation to serve as a collaborator on the project.

## Opinion Leaders

Opinion, or expert, leaders help in the change process by convincing their peers to get on board with the initiative. All key groups, such as the ethics committee or legal department, must be informed or engaged in certain projects, to avoid opposition. Opinion leaders are viewed as knowledgeable about the clinical area, are seen as a respected source of information, and are influential within the system. Opinion leaders are usually discipline specific—physicians influence other physicians, pharmacists influence other pharmacists. These individuals possess both content and organizational knowledge and are experts in determining how new practices will affect current practice. In many settings and for many projects, the physician (unit medical director, attending physician, chief of staff) is a key stakeholder who must be involved in some way. Identifying and engaging the key physician might facilitate smoother implementation of the project. The physician might in turn help obtain the cooperation of other physicians and help advocate for the required resources.

## Customers

Customers are the direct recipients of the product or service provided. Customers can be internal or external, and individuals or entities.

**Building Your Team:** Who are the interprofessional staff you will include in your change effort? Do any of the stakeholders pose an actual threat to successful implementation of your project? Who will be the members on your implementation team? Create a grid that identifies the key stakeholders relevant to your proposed practice change recommendations. Then identify the following:

1. Whether each stakeholder is likely to support, oppose, or remain neutral to the proposed changes
2. The level of influence (low, medium, or high level)
3. How the needs of the customer differ and compare to the needs of the stakeholder

# Complex Adaptive System

In chapter 7, you learned that a *complex adaptive system* (CAS) is defined as "a collection of individual agents that have the freedom to act in ways that are not always predictable and whose actions are interconnected such that one agent's actions changes the context for the other agents."[1(pp.312–313)] Each agent's actions influence the context of the system, so understanding the context, culture, and processes of care are vital to successful change in a CAS. Other examples of CASs are biologic (such as an ant colony) and economic (such as the stock market).

There are eight principal properties of CASs that enable us to identify the components and interactions within the system. We will examine each of these and apply some of them to the self-care example from the opening vignette in chapter 4's "Improvement Opportunity" feature (*see* page 51):

1. **Adaptable elements:** In simple systems, machines and components must be changed by external forces; in CASs, the individual elements (whether antibiotic-resistant organisms or groups of people) can change on their own. The elements within a CAS have the internal capacity to change themselves.

## TABLE A-3  Stakeholder Assessment

| Stakeholder Name | Resistant | Skeptical | Neutral | Supportive | Enthusiastic | Issues or Concerns | "Wins" | Action Items/ Strategy to Influence |
|---|---|---|---|---|---|---|---|---|
| | | | | | | | | |
| | | | | | | | | |
| | | | | | | | | |
| | | | | | | | | |
| | | | | | | | | |
| | | | | | | | | |
| | | | | | | | | |
| | | | | | | | | |

2. **Simple rules:** The underlying norms that occur in a system may or may not be written down, but these norms act as rules that guide individual actions. Although usually not lengthy, these rules provide guidance about how to act (and react) in relation to the other agents in the system.

3. **Nonlinear:** Because of interactions with the system, small changes may have very large effects, and large changes may have very small effects. For example, a hospital may initiate a new program with comprehensive training sessions for all its employees. Although this may be a massive effort, very little change might occur. In contrast, what initially seems like a small incident may have a large impact on how people perform their daily work.

4. **Novel:** Continual creativity is inherently part of the system. In a mechanical system such as an assembly line, actions are repetitive and predictable. In a CAS, the agents often try new ways to perform tasks.

5. **Predicting the unpredictable:** Predicting the future is always challenging. For example, the laws and rules that govern the movement of weather are helpful, but the interaction of those elements is complex, so accurate long-term forecasting is difficult. A complex system, such as weather, must be observed and monitored continually. This is the advantage of monitoring data over time, as discussed in Chapter 6. Run charts and statistical process control charts provide continual monitoring and display a degree of predictability in the systems.

6. **Inherently ordered:** Self-organization is a key idea in complexity science. For instance, there are no distinct rules that tell birds how and where to fly within a flock, yet birds are able to maintain a safe distance from one another and travel safely together.

7. **Contextual and embedded:** As we saw in the target diagram in Chapter 4 (page 64), systems exist within systems and relate to other systems. In Chapter 7 we also discussed the importance of context and culture in a system for identifying the underlying elements that influence the functioning of the system. Although it is possible to identify the individual parts of a CAS, the reductionist approach is not as helpful as considering the fundamental wholeness of the system.

8. **Coevolving:** The seven elements just described all contribute to a CAS moving forward through constant tension and then achieving a new balance. As a system is perturbed by change, the system achieves a new steady state. This holds true for single-celled organisms and also for large health care organizations. The tension, uncertainty, and anxiety that come with change are considered healthy elements in complex systems to achieve greater performance.

## Reference

1. Plsek P. Appendix B: Redesigning health care with insights from the science of complex adaptive systems. In Institute of Medicine: *Crossing the Quality Chasm: A New Health System for the 21st Century.* Washington, DC: National Academy Press, 2001, 309–322.

## Time Line

The creation of a time line is an important step in a quality improvement project. It forces the improvement team to consider when each of the steps might happen. Often, this is a reality check for the team. Team members may want to have their improvement completed in two or three months, but by making a time line, they realize that the necessary steps will require several more months. The time line can help decrease frustration, keep a team on track, and be modified as the work progresses. Either a Gantt chart format or a linear format will work. See Figure A-2 on page 169 for some non–health care examples.

## Communication Plan

A communication plan will contribute to the success of your project. It helps you develop a strategy to communicate with various audiences about your project by identifying the appropriate timing, media (face-to-face meeting, e-mail, and so forth), accountability, message, and follow-up for each opportunity.

To create a communication plan, have the team brainstorm audiences who need to know more about your change initiative. Then for each audience, identify your message and goal (that is, what you're trying to communicate and what you want the audience to do with the message), as well as how you'll get it done (that is, the media, timing, and person responsible for each opportunity). Choose the appropriate media depending on the message you're trying to get across and what you want the recipients to do with the message.

See Tables A-4, A-5, and A-6 on pages 170–172 for two sample templates and an example of a communication plan for a project aiming to reduce emergency room visits.

## FIGURE A-2   Time Line

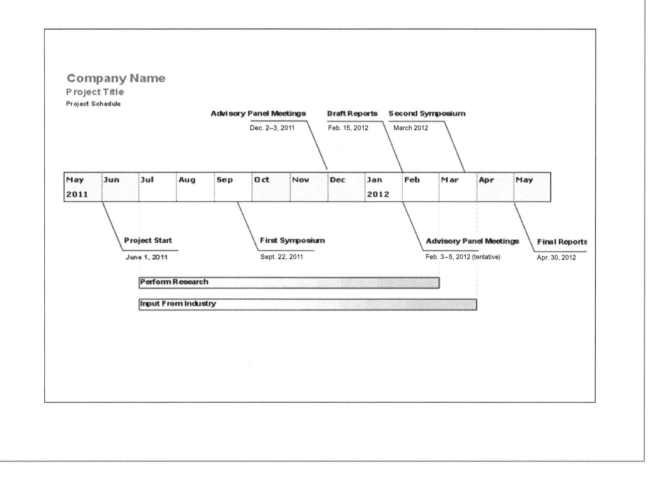

| Activity | March 2013 | April 2013 | May 2013 | June 2013 | July 2013 | August 2013 | September 2013 | October 2013 | November 2013 | December 2013 | January 2014 | February 2014 | Mar 201 |
|---|---|---|---|---|---|---|---|---|---|---|---|---|---|
| Identifying stakeholders | | | | | | | | | | | | | |
| Preintervention workshops | | | | | | | | | | | | | |
| Formation of core group in each cluster | | | | | | | | | | | | | |
| Interventions in community | | | | | | | | | | | | | |
| Process evaluation | | | | | | | | | | | | | |

*Gray shades indicate the time period during which the activity took place.*

**Company Name**
Project Title
Project Schedule

Advisory Panel Meetings — Dec. 2–3, 2011

Draft Reports — Feb. 15, 2012

Second Symposium — March 2012

| May 2011 | Jun | Jul | Aug | Sep | Oct | Nov | Dec | Jan 2012 | Feb | Mar | Apr | May |

Project Start — June 1, 2011

First Symposium — Sept. 22, 2011

Advisory Panel Meetings — Feb. 3–5, 2012 (tentative)

Final Reports — Apr. 30, 2012

Perform Research

Input From Industry

**Communication Matrix**

| Timing | Media | | Audience | | | | Who communicated | What was communicated? | Follow-up and next meeting |
|---|---|---|---|---|---|---|---|---|---|
| | Team meeting (student) | Team meeting (hospital) | Sponsor | Team coach | Process owner | Customer | | | |
| Week 2 | | | | | | | | | |
| Week 3 | | | | | | | | | |
| Week 4 | | | | | | | | | |
| Week 5 | | | | | | | | | |

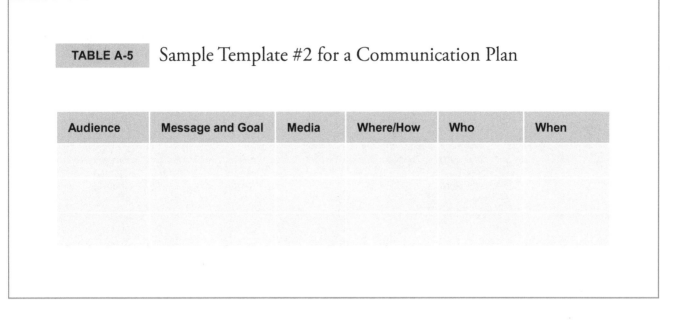

| Audience | Message and Goal | Media | Where/How | Who | When |
|----------|------------------|-------|-----------|-----|------|
|          |                  |       |           |     |      |

**TABLE A-5** Sample Template #2 for a Communication Plan

# Flowchart or Process Map

A flowchart—also known as a process map—visually represents the sequence of steps in a process. Understanding the process as it currently operates is an important step in developing ideas about how to improve it. This makes flowcharts particularly useful in the early phases of improvement work, and then again at its conclusion before closing out the project.

The Institute for Healthcare Improvement has a Quality Improvement Essentials Toolkit[1] that has many essential tools, including how to create a flowchart. (Free registration is required to get access to the tools.) Here are specific benefits of a flowchart:

- Helps identify all the steps in a process by using standard symbols and arrows (*see* Figure A-3, page 173)
- Helps to illustrate redundant steps
- Highlights differences in the process among individuals/ groups
- Can be used to describe the current process or design the new process
- Can show the changes between an "old" and a "new" process
- Can be used as an educational tool when describing the new process
- Can help identify bottlenecks and problem areas

# Cause-and-Effect Diagram

A cause-and-effect diagram—also known as an Ishikawa or fishbone diagram—is a graphic tool used to explore and display the possible causes of a certain effect or identify relationships for potential process improvement (*see* Figure A-4, page 174). Use the classic fishbone diagram when causes group naturally under specific categories (traditionally materials, methods, equipment, environment, and people), or use a process-type cause-and-effect diagram to show causes of problems at each step in the process.

A cause-and-effect diagram has a variety of benefits:
- It helps teams understand that there are many causes that contribute to an effect.
- It graphically displays the relationship of the causes to the effect and to each other.
- It helps to identify areas for improvement.

Here are specific instructions for a cause-and-effect diagram[1]:
- Identify an outcome or effect that you want to study.
- Use either a positive or a negative framework.
  - What elements contribute to good patient satisfaction? (positive framework)
  - What are the causes of poor patient satisfaction? (negative framework)
  - Regardless of which framework is used, the causes and effects must correlate (for example, if the effect is stated in the negative, then the identified causes should be what contributes to that negative cause and not what may make the negative cause go away).

Sample Template #3 for a Communication Plan

| Communication Type | Objective of Communication | Medium | Frequency | Audience | Owner | Deliverable |
|---|---|---|---|---|---|---|
| Kickoff Meeting | Introduce teams to project. Review project objectives and previous work. | Face to face | Once | Project Manager; Project Sponsor; Project Teams | Project Manager | Completed –Agenda –Minutes |
| Project Team Meetings | Review status of project team. | Face to face; conference calls; e-mail | Weekly at minimum | Project Team | Project Manager | Ongoing –Agenda –Minutes |
| Technical Design Meetings | Discuss and develop technical/ design solutions; (for example, data collection methods). | Face to face | As needed | Project Team | Project Team Lead | Ongoing –Agenda –Minutes |
| Project Status Reports | Report on the status of the project, including activities, progress, and issues. | E-mail; conference calls | Biweekly | Project Manager; Project Team | Project Manager | Ongoing –Agenda –Minutes –Project Schedule |
| Monthly Project Status Meetings, Local | Report on the status of the project to local COE group; Project Manager, All Project Teams. | Face to face | Monthly | Project Manager; Project Teams | Project Manager | Ongoing –Agenda –Minutes |
| Monthly Project Status Calls, National | Report on the status. | Conference call | Monthly | Project Managers | Project Manager | –Agenda –Minutes |
| Sponsor Project Status Report | Report on the status of the project to sponsors/ stakeholders. | Face to face/ conference call | Quarterly Sharepoint updates | Project Manager; Sponsors | Project Manager | –Project Status Report –PowerPoint Update Project Schedule |

Flow Chart Symbols

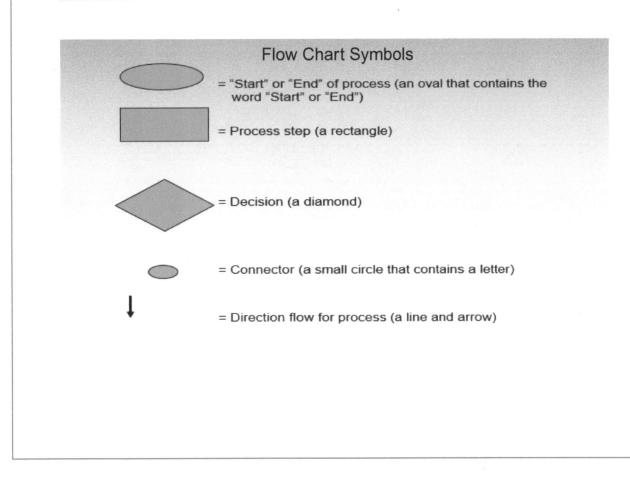

- Brainstorm ideas for possible causes.
- Gather data from the frontline workers and stakeholders.
- Review list of potential causes.
- Eliminate/combine any duplicate causes.
- Identify some general categories for the listed items such as by causes, by characteristics (such as accuracy, courtesy, proficiency, ease of use, time), or according to issues associated with the various steps of the process (from start to finish).
- Review the list and identify which category best describes the item.
- Draw a blank cause-and-effect diagram.
- Fill in the "Cause" and the "Effect" categories.
- List the ideas on the diagram under the appropriate cause category.
- Prioritize causal factors to direct further action.

## Tips for Developing a Survey and Collecting Real-time Data

In quality improvement, it is important to get data from stakeholders, which can be achieved though surveys given to small samples. Improvement teams can develop a "just-in-time" survey and interview patients concurrently. To do this, the team first identifies the decisions that need to be made based on survey outcomes and identifies the survey purpose. Then the team develops survey questions designed to obtain the data needed.

When developing a customized survey, the basic steps include the following:

- Identify the population (for example, congestive heart failure patients).

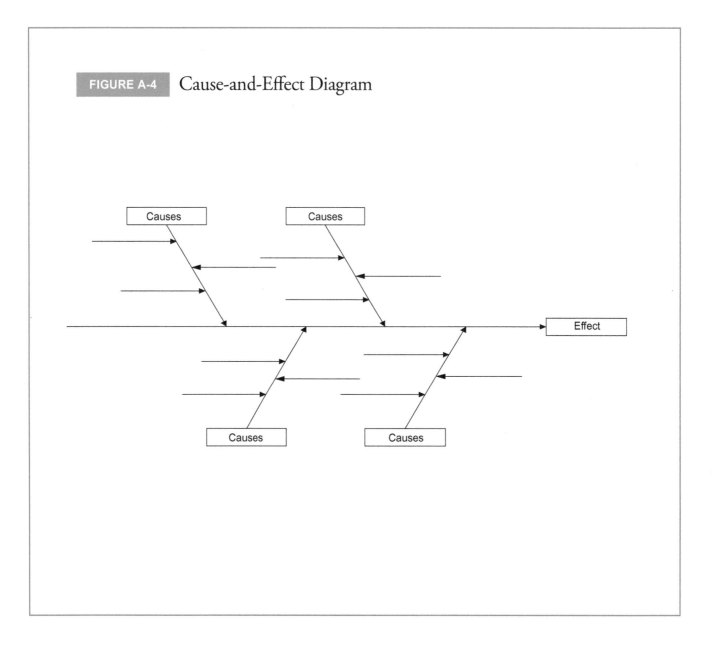

**FIGURE A-4** Cause-and-Effect Diagram

- Identify patients who meet required demographics (that is, patients of specific programs).
- Create a survey process.
- Create a survey scale (for example, 5-point or 10-point).
- Develop survey questions.
- Develop directions for survey completion.

Tips for survey development include the following:
- Develop a short one-page survey that takes 5 minutes or less to complete.
- Focus each question on a single concept. For example, if you want to know if someone is satisfied with turnaround time and promptness, ask it in two separate questions.
- Use visual analogue scales to enhance ease of response.

- Make certain the education level of the question is comparable to the education level of those who will be completing the surveys. The standard education level of lay people is approximately sixth grade.
- Ask for the same type of feedback in several questions. It is one way to measure consistency in responses.
- Consider the wording of survey questions, the order of questions on the survey, the grouping of questions on the survey, the instructions, and the scale type (for example, Strongly Agree to Strongly Disagree).
- Pilot test the survey with four or five stakeholders before administering.
- Based on your pilot outcomes, identify which questions required clarification, were difficult to understand, were left incomplete, and generally led to confusion.

When developing the directions for survey completion, keep the following in mind:

- Include who is to be surveyed.
- Define exclusion criteria—those who will not be surveyed for various reasons, such as comatose patients with no family to interview.
- Specify how the survey process is carried out (concurrent interviews, retrospectively, etc).
- Explain how it will be randomized.
- Identify methods to increase your return rate.

# Change Concepts Worksheet

After reflecting on your flowchart (process flow) and the cause-and-effect diagram (facilitators and barriers), consider the change strategies in Table A-7, below. Change strategies are used to identify potential changes to test with Plan–Do–Study–Act. Like many of these tools, the strategies are for brainstorming to consider broadly the possible changes that may be effective.

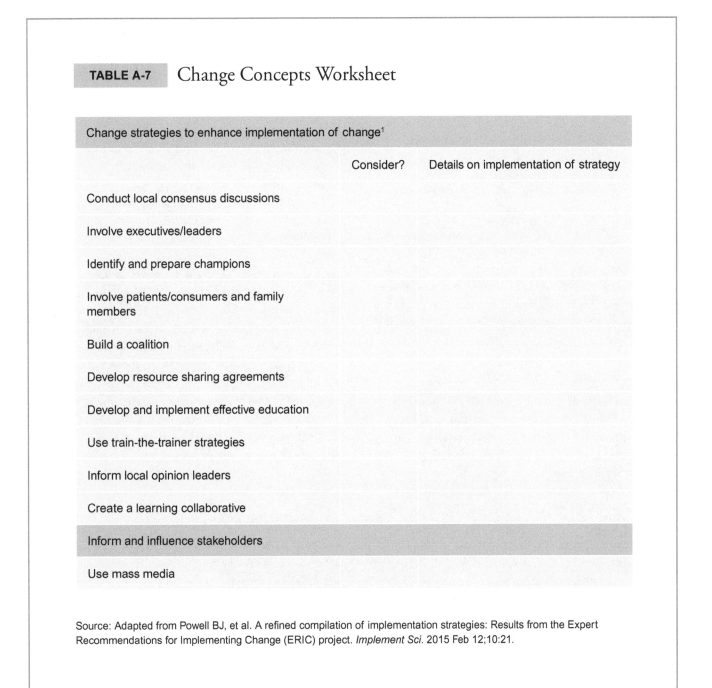

**TABLE A-7**    Change Concepts Worksheet

| Change strategies to enhance implementation of change[1] | | |
|---|---|---|
| | Consider? | Details on implementation of strategy |
| Conduct local consensus discussions | | |
| Involve executives/leaders | | |
| Identify and prepare champions | | |
| Involve patients/consumers and family members | | |
| Build a coalition | | |
| Develop resource sharing agreements | | |
| Develop and implement effective education | | |
| Use train-the-trainer strategies | | |
| Inform local opinion leaders | | |
| Create a learning collaborative | | |
| **Inform and influence stakeholders** | | |
| Use mass media | | |

Source: Adapted from Powell BJ, et al. A refined compilation of implementation strategies: Results from the Expert Recommendations for Implementing Change (ERIC) project. *Implement Sci*. 2015 Feb 12;10:21.

# Plan–Do–Study–Act (PDSA) Worksheet

The Plan–Do–Study–Act (PDSA) cycle can be used to document a test of change. Running a PDSA cycle is another way of saying testing a change—you develop a plan to test the change (Plan); carry out the test (Do); observe, analyze, and learn from the test (Study); and determine what modifications, if any, to make for the next cycle (Act).

In most improvement projects, teams will test several different changes, and each change may go through several PDSA cycles as you continue to learn. Fill out one PDSA worksheet for each change you test. Keep a file (either electronic or hard copy) of all PDSA cycles for all the changes your team tests.

The Institute for Healthcare Improvement Quality Improvement Essentials Toolkit provides an example of another PDSA worksheet (*see* Table A-8, page 177).[1]

# Team Evaluation

Many team assessment tools can be used during your improvement work. The main purpose is to get feedback on group dynamics to identify what is going well and what is not going well. Team evaluation is one tool that can help a team assess how it is functioning and what might help it function better.

### Goals, Roles, Processes, and Interpersonal (GRPI) Analysis Tool

The Goals, Roles, Processes, and Interpersonal (GRPI) Analysis allows each team member to express his or her perception on how well the team is functioning in several important ways (*see* Figure A-5, page 178). In many cases, team members' perceptions may be different, which provides a great starting point to discuss how things are going. Ask team members to evaluate the effectiveness of the team by ranking their own perceptions of the goals, roles, processes, and interpersonal relationships. (It may be helpful to ask team members to do this in advance of a team meeting—submitting their ratings anonymously to an impartial facilitator who can post the results at a team meeting and facilitate a discussion.) Discuss the results and what they mean for the effectiveness of the group. Consider what changes need to be made to help the team function better.

# Creating a Storyboard

Storyboarding is a highly visible process of gathering, evaluating, and organizing information that has become an important tool for planning and visualizing work. It can be used for displaying or for sharing the results of an improvement project. For publishing your quality improvement work, the first part of Chapter 9 describes the Standards for Quality Improvement Reporting Excellence (SQUIRE) publication guidelines.[1] SQUIRE can help you be more successful in publishing your improvement work.

There are many ways to create a storyboard, but most effective storyboards use a combination of narrative and images. When using storyboarding to tell the story of an improvement project, keep the following in mind:

- Determine how the team wants to depict the progress and the improvements made during the process improvement project.
- Organize the board to highlight different tools used in various stages to plan, define, analyze, and improve the process problem.
- Include graphic or visual representations that can tell the story or the outcome of the project without much explanation.

Here are two examples. The first is from the US Department of Veterans Affairs (VA) Cleveland Louis Stokes VA Center of Excellence in Primary Care (*see* Figure A-6, page 179). This storyboard depicts the resident physicians' work to analyze and reduce pain in the emergency department. The details in the storyboard are less important than the layout. Notice the headers that are used and the flow of information in three of the columns. The storyboard has a clear focus on the aim of the work, the methods and changes that were made, and the data. The data take up a large portion of the right-hand column. This is appropriate, as viewers of a storyboard will be interested in the data.

The second storyboard is from the White River Junction VA Hospital in Vermont (*see* Figure A-7, page 180). It depicts the work of a team of resident physicians who worked to improve counseling for tobacco cessation for patients admitted to the hospital. Notice the list of "major" PDSA cycles in the lower left-hand column. When creating a storyboard, you need to focus your message. It may not be possible to share everything that happened during the improvement work, so the team is sharing only the major

## TABLE A-8    PDSA Worksheet

DESCRIBE the intervention you would like to implement:

| # | PLAN | Description | Facilitators | Barriers | STUDY | |
|---|------|-------------|--------------|----------|-------|---|
| | STAKEHOLDERS (administrators, peers, other professionals) | | | | Was your prediction accurate? | Yes    No |
| | PEOPLE involved in the process | | | | What did you observe that was not part of the plan? | |
| | COMMUNICATION STRATEGY | | | | Was the cycle carried out as planned? | |
| | SCOPE: | | | | | |
| | SCALE: | | | | | |
| | **DO** | | | | **ACT** | |
| | Who is the person responsible? | | | | What are the next steps to improve this PDSA? | |
| | When done | | | | | |
| | Where done | | | | What is the next PDSA? | |
| | How done | | | | | |
| | Data collection | | | | | |

**Source:** Institute for Healthcare Improvement. Tools: Plan-Do-Study-Act (PDSA) Worksheet. 2017. Accessed Nov 27, 2017. http://www.ihi.org/resources/Pages/Tools/PlanDoStudyActWorksheet.aspx.

| **FIGURE A-5** | GRPI (Goals, Roles, Processes, and Interpersonal) Analysis |

| Rate the Team's Effectiveness | Low | | | | High |
|---|---|---|---|---|---|
| **GOALS** – How clear and in agreement are we on the mission and goals of our team and projects? | 1 | 2 | 3 | 4 | 5 |
| **ROLES** – How well do we understand, agree on, and fulfill the roles and responsibilities for our team? | 1 | 2 | 3 | 4 | 5 |
| **PROCESSES** – How well do we understand and agree on the way in which we'll approach our project and our team? | 1 | 2 | 3 | 4 | 5 |
| **INTERPERSONAL** – How well are the relationships on our team working? How open, trusting, and accountable are we? | 1 | 2 | 3 | 4 | 5 |

Other areas we need to discuss: _____

_____

_____

PDSA cycles. This poster also includes a control chart annotated with the PDSA cycles and an acknowledgement of an important team member.

## Reference

1. Ogrinc G, et al. SQUIRE 2.0 (Standards for QUality Improvement Reporting Excellence): Revised publication guidelines from a detailed consensus process. *BMJ Qual Saf.* 2016 Dec;25(12):986–992.

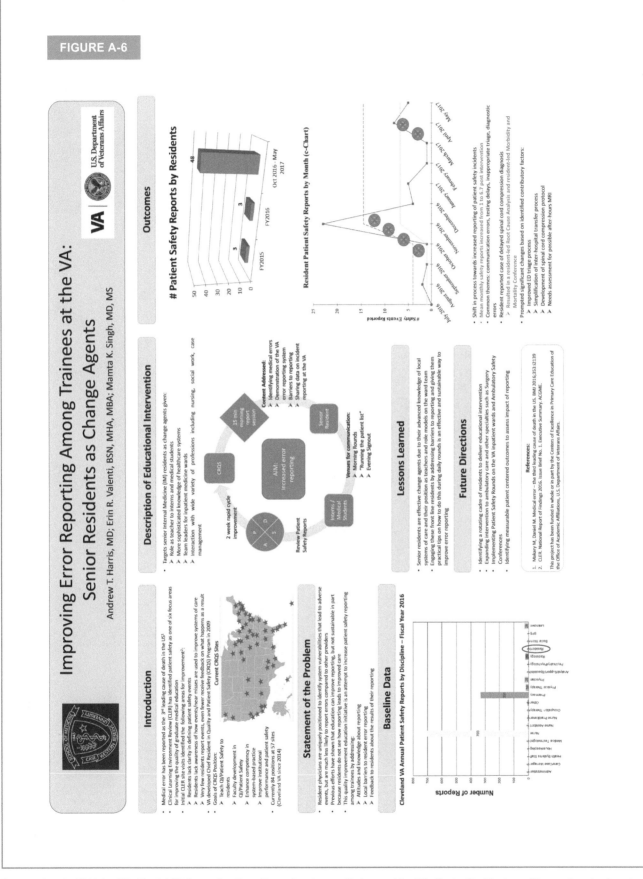

**Source:** Harris AT, Valenti E, Singh MK. Improving Error Reporting Among Trainees at the VA: Senior Residents as Change Agents. American Association of Medical Colleges (AAMC) Integrating Quality Meeting. Chicago, IL. June 2017. Printed with permission.

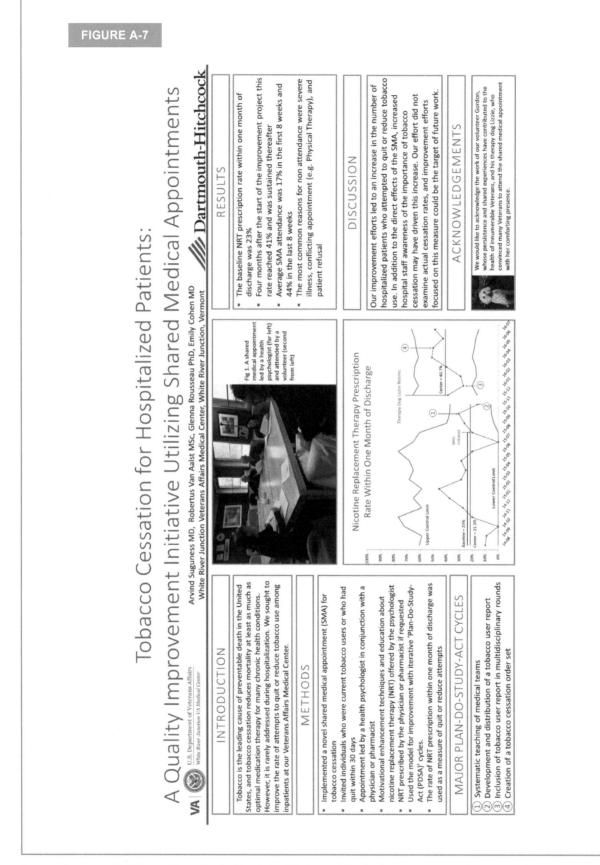

# Tobacco Cessation for Hospitalized Patients:
## A Quality Improvement Initiative Utilizing Shared Medical Appointments

Arvind Suguness MD, Robertus Van Aalst MSc, Glenna Rousseau PhD, Emily Cohen MD
White River Junction Veterans Affairs Medical Center, White River Junction, Vermont

### INTRODUCTION

Tobacco is the leading cause of preventable death in the United States, and tobacco cessation reduces mortality at least as much as optimal medication therapy for many chronic health conditions. However, it is rarely addressed during hospitalization. We sought to improve the rate of attempts to quit or reduce tobacco use among inpatients at our Veterans Affairs Medical Center.

### METHODS

- Implemented a novel shared medical appointment (SMA) for tobacco cessation
- Invited individuals who were current tobacco users or who had quit within 30 days
- Appointment led by a health psychologist in conjunction with a physician or pharmacist
- Motivational enhancement techniques and education about nicotine replacement therapy (NRT) offered by the psychologist
- NRT prescribed by the physician or pharmacist if requested
- Used the model for improvement with iterative 'Plan-Do-Study-Act (PDSA)' cycles.
- The rate of NRT prescription within one month of discharge was used as a measure of quit or reduce attempts

### MAJOR PLAN-DO-STUDY-ACT CYCLES

1. Systematic teaching of medical teams
2. Development and distribution of a tobacco user report
3. Inclusion of tobacco user report in multidisciplinary rounds
4. Creation of a tobacco cessation order set

Fig 1. A shared medical appointment led by a health psychologist (far left) and attended by a volunteer (second from left)

Nicotine Replacement Therapy Prescription Rate Within One Month of Discharge

### RESULTS

- The baseline NRT prescription rate within one month of discharge was 23%
- Four months after the start of the improvement project this rate reached 41% and was sustained thereafter
- Average SMA attendance was 17% in the first 8 weeks and 44% in the last 8 weeks
- The most common reasons for non attendance were severe illness, conflicting appointment (e.g. Physical Therapy), and patient refusal

### DISCUSSION

Our improvement efforts led to an increase in the number of hospitalized patients who attempted to quit or reduce tobacco use. In addition to the direct effects of the SMA, increased hospital staff awareness of the importance of tobacco cessation may have driven this increase. Our effort did not examine actual cessation rates, and improvement efforts focused on this measure could be the target of future work.

### ACKNOWLEDGEMENTS

We would like to acknowledge the work of our volunteer Gordon, whose persistence and shared experiences have contributed to the health of innumerable Veterans, and his therapy dog Lizzie, who convinced many Veterans to attend the shared medical appointment with her comforting presence.

**Source:** Suguness AL. Tobacco Cessation for Hospitalized Patients: A Quality Improvement Initiative Utilizing Shared Medical Appointments. Poster presented at: American College of Physicians Annual Meeting; May, 2017; San Diego, CA. Printed with permission.

# Index

# G

# H

# I

# M

in Model for Improvement, 21–23, 40, 111,
112, 121
monitoring and tracking of, 123
phases of, 121–122
successive cycles over time, 122, 124, 125
in system changes, 119–125, 127
worksheet on, 176, 177
Plan phase of PDSA cycle, 121, 123
Pneumonia
community-acquired, 25–26, 32
ventilator-associated, 89–91
Polar-area diagram, 68, 69
Potassium serum levels after CABG surgery, lab
turnaround times for, 104–107
Preventive care
creating aim statement on, 44
evidence-based practice and improvement in,
42, 44
identified as focus for improvement, 39–40, 42
Privacy of health information, 49
Process analysis, 7, 51–65
arrogance and illiteracy in, 52
on clinic visits. *See* Clinic visits, process analysis
on culture, context, and systems factors in, 57,
60–64
in fall risk reduction, 116, 117, 119
importance of, 52–53
measures in, 53, 80
methods of, 53–60
model created in, 53
in Model for Improvement, 65
study questions on, 65
in system changes, 115, 116, 117, 119
terminology related to, 52
Proficiency in quality improvement, 156, 157
Prospective cohort studies, 32
Published reports on improvement efforts
compared to research reports, 142
context section of, 142, 144, 146
rationale section of, 142, 143, 145–146
SQUIRE guidelines on, 8, 142–150, 176
study of intervention section in, 144, 145, 146
summary section of, 147
PubMed, 33, 36
Pyramid diagram on strength of evidence, 31

# Q

Qualitative data, 71, 81
Quality and Safety Education for Nurses, 154
Quality gaps, 7, 12–14, 24
in beta blocker use after myocardial infarction,
13, 22–23
identifying improvement areas in, 41
Quality improvement activities. *See* Improvement
activities
Quantitative data, 71, 81–82
Questions asked in evidence-based practice and
improvement, 29–30

# R

Randomized controlled trials, 31, 32, 33
Rapid response teams in cardiac arrest, 141–142
Rationale section in quality improvement reporting,
142, 143, 145–146
Readiness for change, 125–126, 164–165
Reference librarian assistance in literature searches,
33–36
Relevancy of improvement project, 43–44
Replication of results, 91
probability statistics in, 91
Research
in continuum with quality improvement and
patient care, 43, 45, 49
differentiated from improvement activities, 147,
148–150
for evidence-based practice and improvement,
25–36
IRB review of, 43, 44
literature searches in, 33–36
measurement for, 72, 73, 74, 76
publishing results of, 142
Resistance to change, 125
Retrospective cohort studies, 32
Robust Process Improvement (RPI), 16, 21, 22
Rogers, Everett, 114, 115, 134
Role-modeling quality improvement in educational
processes, 153–154
Run charts, 8, 89, 91, 104
on beta blockers in heart failure, 99, 100–101
on candy distribution, 97, 98
common-cause variations in, 99, 101
compared to control charts, 94–95
components of, 91, 92

System of health care
    compared to individual patient care, 12, 16, 17
    as complex adaptive system, 112–113, 166–168
    in continuum with individual patient care, 41
    definition of, 63
    leader of, on improvement team, 19
    levels of, 63–64
    making changes in. *See* System changes
    as pillar in quality improvement, 17, 18

# T

Teach-back method
    in discharge instructions, 129–130
    in hypertension management, 113, 126
Teaching quality improvement, 8, 147, 150–154
Teaching status of hospitals, and beta blocker use in
    myocardial infarction, 12–13
Team approach
    in cardiac arrest rapid response, 141–142
    in myocardial infarction care, 12, 14
    in patient rounds, 25, 67–68
    in quality improvement. *See* Improvement teams
Theoretical limit of performance, 46
Time line in improvement projects, 168, 169
Tools for improvement activities, 8, 159–180
Training. *See* Education and training
Transportation (work flow) diagram, 54, 57–58, 61
Trip Database, 33, 34, 35

# U

Unfiltered information, strength of evidence in,
    31–32
University of Colorado Hospital, evidence-based
    practice in, 26, 27, 29
Upper control limit, 91, 93, 96, 105, 107

# V

Value equation, 79–80, 83
Variation, 74–76
    common-cause. *See* Common-cause variation
    indications for action in, 94, 96
    in run charts, 95–96, 99, 101
    special-cause. *See* Special-cause variation
    in statistical process control charts, 91
Ventilator-associated pneumonia, 89–91
Veterans Affairs hospitals, 43–44
    storyboards in, 176, 179–180

# W

Work flow diagrams, 54, 57–58, 61

# X

XmR control charts, 91, 93, 96, 97–107
    on beta blockers in heart failure, 102–104, 105
    on candy distribution, 97, 98, 99
    on diabetes management, 84
    on fall rate, 116, 121, 122
    on lab turnaround times for potassium results,
    106–107